A SENSORY MOTOR APPROACH TO FEEDING

LORI L. OVERLAND,
M.S., CCC-SLP, C/NDT

ROBYN MERKEL-WALSH,
M.A., CCC-SLP

Copyright © 2013 by TalkTools®
TalkTools®
1852 Wallace School Road, Suite H
Charleston, South Carolina 29407

All rights reserved. No part of this book may be kept in an information storage or retrieval system, transmitted or reproduced in any form or by any means without prior written permission of the Publisher.

Library of Congress Cataloging in Publication Data 2013950228

ISBN 978-1-932460-07-0

Cover Image: Patrick Sweeney Photography
Cover Design and Book Layout: Lauren J. Kendall
Photography Credits: Patrick Sweeney Photography, Deborah K. O'Brien
Illustrations: Lauren J. Kendall, Pogostickstudio.com

IN LOVING MEMORIES OF OUR MOTHERS
RONNI SCHWARTZ FRANKEL
AND LOUISE LAWLER DERISO

TABLE OF CONTENTS

ABOUT THE AUTHORS

FOREWORD AND ACKNOWLEDGMENTS

CHAPTER 1: 1
A SENSORY MOTOR APPROACH TO FEEDING

CHAPTER 2: 11
THE ORAL PHASE OF FEEDING

CHAPTER 3: 23
FACTORS THAT INFLUENCE FEEDING

CHAPTER 4: 41
NUTRITIONAL CONCERNS

CHAPTER 5: 61
SENSORY PROCESSING - A SIMPLIFIED SUMMARY

CHAPTER 6: 69
ASSESSMENT

CHAPTER 7: 87
A PRE-FEEDING PROGRAM

CHAPTER 8: 113
SENSORY BASED DIET SHAPING

CHAPTER 9: 127
THERAPEUTIC FEEDING

CHAPTER 10: 167
WRITING A PROGRAM PLAN

APPENDIX A: 197
GLUTEN-FREE, CASEIN-FREE DIET

APPENDIX B: 201
ORAL SENSORY-MOTOR COOKBOOK

APPENDIX C: 209
NUTRITIONAL CHARTS AND GUIDELINES

APPENDIX D: 211
FORMS

APPENDIX E: 233
SAMPLE REPORT

REFERENCES 243

ABOUT THE AUTHORS

Lori L. Overland, M.S., CCC-SLP, C/NDT is a speech and language pathologist with more than 33 years of professional experience.

Lori specializes in dealing with the unique needs of infants, toddlers, pre-schoolers and school-aged children with oral motor, feeding, and speech disorders. She has received an award from the Connecticut Down Syndrome Association for her work within this population.

Lori consults with children from all over the world, providing evaluations, re-evaluations, program plans, and week-long therapy programs. Lori also provides consults to local school districts and Birth-to-Three organizations. Her goal in addressing feeding and speech challenges is to improve the quality of life for both the children she serves and their families.

In addition to her private practice, Lori is a member of TalkTools® speakers bureau. Lori has lectured on sensory motor feeding disorders across the United States and internationally. Her classes, "Feeding Therapy: A Sensory-Motor Approach" and "Developing Oral-Motor Feeding Skills in the Down Syndrome Population" are approved for ASHA and AOTA CEUs.

Lori is the author of *A Sensory-Motor Approach to Feeding*, "Perspectives on Swallowing and Swallowing Disorders (Dysphagia)" (October 2011) and "Food for Thought," *Advance Magazine for Occupational Therapists* (May 2001).

She holds degrees from Hofstra University and Adelphi University, and has her neurodevelopmental certification.

Robyn Merkel-Walsh MA, CCC-SLP is a Licensed Speech Pathologist with over 19 years of experience in the state of NJ. She is employed full time by the Ridgefield Board of Education and runs a private practice in Ridgefield, NJ.

Robyn specializes in Oral-Placement and myofunctional disorders in children. Her private practice focuses on Oral-Placement disorders in children, particularly those within the autism spectrum. She conducts evaluations and Program Plans for children across the tri-state area. Her publications include *SMILE (Systematic Intervention for Lingual Elevation)*, Art Talk, Handy Handouts, *OPTS Kit*, and she co-authored *Sensory Stix* and *OPT Goals for Speech Clarity*. She has also written several articles for the TalkTools® website, and *Advance Magazine for Speech Pathologists*.

Robyn is a lecturer for professional enhancement courses as part of TalkTools® speakers bureau. She teaches ASHA CE-approved Tongue Thrust and Autism classes, and has been invited to speak on Oral Placement disorders by the New Milford Board of Education, the Apraxia Network, AAPPSPA, and the MOSAIC Foundation. She is actively involved in parental support groups for apraxia and autism, and monitors an interactive Oral Placement Discussion Board on Facebook. Robyn was a chief clinician in a research project for the Moebius Foundation, and trains TalkTools® Level 3 and 4 candidates.

Robyn received both her undergraduate and graduate degrees from Montclair State University, where she was later invited to be an adjunct/clinical supervisor. She has also taught classes at Bergen Community College, and is a former clinical site coordinator for Seton Hall University. She is a member of ASHA, NJSHA, the NJEA, the Bergen County Apraxia Association and is a former member of the International Association of Oralfacial Myology.

Robyn has specialized training in Oral-Placement Disorders, feeding, apraxia, Applied Behavioral Analysis, autism, cranio-facial anomalies, Beckman Techniques, and PROMPT. Robyn also has a specialized interest in integrative medicine and holistic healing.

PREFACE AND ACKNOWLEDGMENTS

FROM LORI: When a member of a family has a feeding disorder it impacts every member of the family and all aspects of life. Family members struggle to get through the day as they attempt to insure their loved one gets adequate nutrition.

Most of us live to eat! Food is life! Our daily meals provide enjoyment beyond the physical experience. They are opportunities to interact and share with members of our families. Social outings with friends frequently involve food. Holidays and life cycle events are planned around meals.

Many of our clients eat just enough to stay alive. They do not have the underlying sensory motor skills to handle food. They may compromise their respiratory systems and safety when they eat. They have often self-limited their diets based upon their sensory and motor systems. Food is not innately reinforcing, and mealtime is often stressful.

There are feeding clinics across the country and throughout the world that address medical and behavioral issues related to feeding disorders. In addition, there are numerous books that address the structures and functions to support feeding, medical issues associated with feeding, food exploration, and behavioral interventions. Few programs address the underlying interaction of the sensory and motor systems as a primary concern in the feeding paradigm.

This is a book about developing the oral sensory motor skills to support feeding. The underlying premise of this book is simple. As therapists we must be able to task analyze the sensory motor skills needed for safe, nutritive feeding. Our evaluations must take into consideration our client's medical, respiratory, and postural issues. However, if our clients present with compromised oral sensory motor skills, our therapy must have strategies for developing these motor skills.

For the past 32 years, I have worked with infants, toddlers, preschool children, and school age children with a wide range of diagnoses.

The techniques shared in this book are not specific to any age group or diagnosis. They have been used from birth through geriatrics. As a working therapist, I know it is impossible to ever know "everything." I believe we are "bag ladies" (and gentlemen). We carry our "bags" of knowledge and experience with us, and dig deep when we work with challenging clients. These strategies are among those in my "bag". I will always be grateful to those therapists from whom I have had the opportunity to learn over the years.

My deepest gratitude goes to my friend and mentor Sara Rosenfeld-Johnson who, twenty-four years ago, taught me to be a good observer, and to task analyze the motor skills for feeding and speech. Sara challenged me to be creative with this knowledge. For the past fifteen years Sara has encouraged (*begged, pleaded, threatened, etc.*) me to write this book.

I will be eternally grateful (and so will Sara) to Robyn Walsh, who made this happen. Robyn is an amazing therapist and an even better friend. Robyn specializes in working with children on the Autism spectrum. Her vast expertise in nutritional issues with this population and behavior management added additional dimensions to this book. Thank you to the TalkTools® team: Renee Roy Hill, Lisa Brideson Glynn, Emilia DelPino, Louisa Wong, and of course Sara and Robyn, for using these techniques and providing ongoing feedback over the years. Robyn and I would like to offer a special thanks to Diane Bahr for reading the manuscript for this book, and sharing her knowledge and expertise. To my assistant and good friend Debbie Ripperger, thank you for always keeping me organized and always being one step ahead of me.

To the children and families who I have been privileged to work with over the last 32 years ... thank you for inviting me to be part of your lives and for trusting me to join you on this journey. You have taught me more than any therapist, book, or class.

Last but certainly not least, I owe thanks to my wonderful and always supportive husband, Keith, and my incredible children, Scott, Jamie, and Randy. The learning always started at home! I love you all more than you will ever know!

I hope this book will be added to your "bag" and will be well used in your journey to provide services to the children and families you are privileged to serve.

FROM ROBYN: It was over twenty years ago that I first took a TalkTools® class in New Jersey. As a graduate student, my eyes were opened by my amazing speech therapist/aunt, Janine McGovern-Lawler. I knew at the very beginning of my career that I wanted to dedicate my clinic to (what was then called) oral motor therapy.

As my career has evolved, I have become more involved with feeding therapy. Working in an autism program, and with many children on the spectrum, I have taken a great interest in the connection between the diet and autism. As Lori stated, some of these children eat just to survive. Feeding therapy is such a critical component of being a speech –language pathologist. I have taken numerous hours of course work on feeding, but I have not met a therapist who has taught me more practical and effective techniques than my dear mentor and friend, Lori Overland. As I have watched her teach over the years I am always delighted to find that whatever Lori teaches me can be done in my clinic the next day to help a child make progress. With her sensory-motor approach to feeding, I have learned how to expand children's diets, and develop their oral sensory-motor skills for both feeding and speech.

When Lori asked me to help her write this book I was both flattered and afraid! How could I possibly enhance Lori's immense knowledge? As the process developed, I realized that I had more to offer than I originally considered. We met in hotels all across the tri-state area and shared many cups of coffee and glasses of wine to finish this project. I am ecstatic that I was able to add to Lori's "bag." The fact that I was involved in this project is certainly one of my greatest accomplishments.

I would also like to thank the TalkTools® team, especially Sara Rosenfeld-Johnson for taking me under her wing nearly 15 years ago, and bringing out the best in me. Without her, and Lori, I would not be as accomplished as I am today. Many thanks to: Luke Blessinger, Beth Howard, Lauren Kendall, Renee Roy-Hill, Lisa Brideson-Glynn, and all of the therapists pursuing certification, and to those who support our efforts. I would also like to thank my Aunt Janine, who inspired me to become a speech therapist in the first place. Diane Bahr, thanks for your undying efforts to help us with Evidence Based Practice, and for all of your edits to this book. Many thanks to Sarah Murray, my graduate intern, who was wonderful in helping with the APA formatting of this text. Finally, I thank the Ridgefield Board of Education, which has supported me in my research, writing, and learning throughout my career. My first principal, Lawrence Dunn, was the first supervisor to encourage me to write and develop products, and I will be eternally grateful, may he rest in peace.

Lori and I would like to thank the wonderful families who volunteered for photo shoots in both of our office locations. The children are the true stars of this text.

On a personal note, I thank my husband Chris, and my son Jaden, who love me, even though I work the hours of three people. They encourage me to fulfill my dreams, and support all that I do. I love them "more than cupcakes!"

CHAPTER 1:
A SENSORY-MOTOR APPROACH TO FEEDING

LEADING GOALS/POINTS

What is a sensory motor approach to feeding?

What is a pre-feeding program?

What is a therapeutic feeding program?

What is a "sensory-motor" approach to feeding?

The best way to understand a sensory-motor approach to feeding is by example:

Example #1

Imagine smelling freshly popped popcorn. What sensations do you experience? You begin to salivate and reach for a handful. You open your mouth wide enough to accommodate several pieces. Initially, you taste salt and possibly the butter. If these are tastes you enjoy, the sensory feedback is positive. You may think, "I like the way this tastes!" Next, you bite down and experience the crunchy texture. This is another sensory experience that triggers a motor response. It is crunchy. "I can't just swallow it. I have to chew it." So, you move it to the chewing surface in your mouth. For most of us, that is the molar ridge, where your first molars are located. How did you get the popcorn from the front of your mouth to the molar ridge? Most of us use our tongue tip and the lateral borders of the tongue to collect the popcorn and sweep it to our chewing surface. We use the lateral border of the tongue and our cheek to stabilize the chewed popcorn, as we break the food down. How do we know how hard to bite and how long to chew? There is an ongoing interaction between our sensory and motor systems that allows us to determine when it is adequately broken down, and we use sensory feedback to ascertain when the bolus can be swallowed. If we put a lot of popcorn in our mouth, we may lateralize the bolus with our tongue from one molar ridge to the other, and jaw movement is activated to chew the popcorn. When the food is adequately masticated we get sensory feedback to swallow. Your sensory-motor experience was positive. The next time you are offered this food, you recall the smell and taste of popcorn, and are eager to eat.

Example #2

Now imagine that you are offered the very same salty, buttery popcorn. It smells good, and your initial sensory response to the taste is very similar. However, this time you do not have the motor skills to move the popcorn to the molar ridge to chew it. The popcorn sits on the surface of your tongue. You use an immature motor pattern such as a suckle or munch chew to break down the popcorn. The kernels of corn feel rough on the surface of your tongue. You are pooling saliva because of the flavor, but you cannot swallow because of the large pieces sitting on the surface of your tongue. Very quickly, your initial pleasure with the taste turns to discomfort. What am I going to do with this food on my tongue? It is not breaking down. Your jaw and tongue tire. Can you spit it out? Can you swallow it whole? You panic and swallow. The popcorn gets stuck on the back of your tongue. You gag and throw up. The sensory feedback you get is a feeling of panic. You go in to a fright, fight, flight mode. The next time you are offered popcorn you turn away, shut your mouth tightly, and adamantly refuse.

Discussion

Children who have the experience described in Example #2 are often referred to our offices for a feeding consult. Well-meaning parents and therapists have given children food they do not have the sensory-motor skills to handle secondary to one of many of the complications discussed

SAFE, EFFECTIVE, NUTRITIVE FEEDING

in Chapter 3. They have not gone through the "typical" development of oral sensory-motor skills due to medical issues, postural issues, tone issues, or sensory processing issues. Their compensatory motor skills are not adequate to handle the foods they are offered. They have had scary experiences with food. For many of these clients, food refusal is not behavioral, it is adaptive.

For other referrals we receive, what you see in "life" is often what you see in feeding. This is particularly true for the clients with whom we work who are on the autism spectrum or have significant sensory processing issues. Clients who have difficulty with transitions, who have very specific routines for moving through life, will only wear a certain color or type of clothing, and frequently have difficulty with sensory experiences. These individuals often have the same "rules" regarding feeding. They will eat only foods that are a certain color or a certain texture. They may smell everything. They may be willing to put non-food items in their mouths but refuse edible items. They may not be able to tolerate toothbrushing or routine dental exams. Many of these clients "ate everything" when they were infants, yet when they transitioned from purees to solid foods, they refused all but a few foods. Their experiences with solid foods have been self-limited, and they also may not have developed the sensory-motor skills to handle a range of food textures. These issues will be addressed more specifically in Chapter 5. However, they also may have delays in oral sensory motor skill development that need to be addressed before a sensory food exploration or behavioral program is recommended.

What is a pre-feeding program?

The goal of a pre-feeding program is to develop the motor skills to support safe, effective, nutritive feeding. There is a "range" of motor skills that can be judged to be within normal limits for eating. You may observe someone eating who uses compensatory patterns, but has adequate nutrition and speech that is within acceptable limits. A pre-feeding program in this type of case would not be recommended. Pre-feeding activities are for those clients who do not have adequate nutrition and/or have co-existing speech clarity issues. Clients who require a pre-feeding program may have a diagnosis such as: Down syndrome, Moebius, autism, cleft palate, or generalized hypotonia. However, a pre-feeding program may be appropriate for children or adults with a wide range of diagnoses. For the purpose of this text, the concern lies with the observation of sensory-motor functions rather than the differential diagnosis.

Oral stimulation techniques have long been used with infants, toddlers, pre-schoolers, school-aged children and adults with neuromotor disorders (Bahr 2001; Morris & Klein 1987; O'Sullivan 2007; Pierce, 1980; Rocha et al., 2007; Sjögreen et al, 2010; Marshalla, 2012). The goal of these oral sensory programs has reportedly been to prepare the mouth for feeding, to decrease oral defensiveness, or to increase sensory awareness. Input may be provided with a caregiver's gloved hand, a Nuk® brush, or a vibrating probe. Input is often provided in the cheeks, on the surface of the tongue, on the gums etc. (Marshalla, 2007). There is little regard for the motor skills needed to handle foods. The sensory reaction is often fright, fight, and flight. Children can have the same responses to a pre-feeding program as they have had with food. This is why the progression of a pre-feeding program is very important. If the input is uncomfortable or the child is made to gag or vomit, therapy itself can be unsuccessful.

You cannot separate the sensory and motor systems. Whenever

YOU CANNOT SEPARATE THE SENSORY AND MOTOR SYSTEMS

you move you get sensory feedback, and sensory input influences motor development. The mouth is a center for sensory organization. Sensory input can be organizing, or it can be disorganizing. Once again, well-meaning parents and therapists often increase sensory defensiveness in and around the mouth by providing extraneous oral sensory input. Therefore, it is essential to assess the client's current motor skills (see Chapter 6) and task analyze the motor skills they need to handle food (e.g., for: bottle, breast, spoon, solids, cup, or straw).

Your program should start with a motor goal, and sensory input should be mapped onto that motor goal. The "tools" you use (food, a gloved hand, an oral sensory-motor tool such as ARK's Z-Vibe®, Chewy Tube, Toothette, oral massage brush etc.) should be based upon the sensory input your client needs to facilitate the motor skill you are seeking to develop (Bahr & Johnson, 2010).

If you are a parent, and someone has recommended oral sensory input, ask what motor skill is being facilitated to support safe, effective, nutritive feeding. There should be NO EXTRANEOUS ORAL SENSORY INPUT. The goal of a pre-feeding plan is to establish the necessary oral sensory-motor skills for feeding.

What is a therapeutic feeding program?

The goal of a therapeutic feeding program is to develop a set of techniques that support safe feeding and maximize a client's postural stability, muscle tone, sensory processing, and oral sensory-motor skills. Where you put food in the mouth influences what the client will do with that food.

Imagine biting a pretzel stick with your front teeth. Your tongue comes forward to meet the food (Position E).

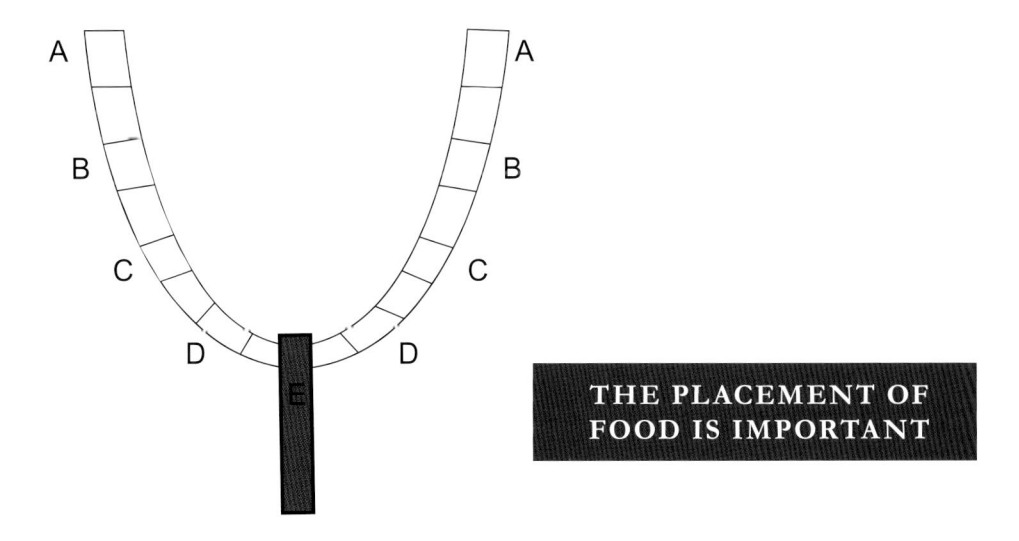

THE PLACEMENT OF FOOD IS IMPORTANT

Now take the same pretzel stick and place it perpendicular to the lateral molar ridge on your first molar (position A):

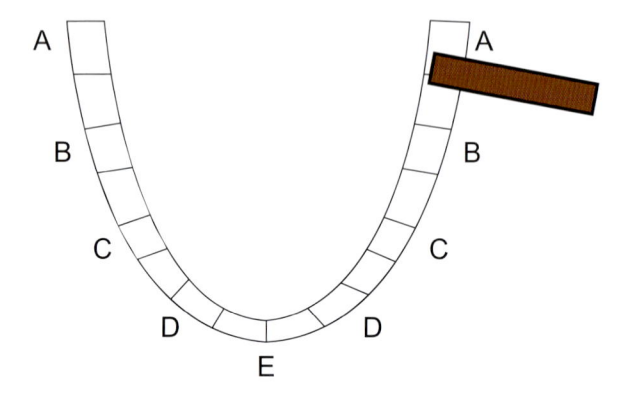

Your tongue should retract and lateralize.

The placement of the food becomes very important for a client with compromised motor skills. For a client who cannot move food to the chewing surface, it will be important to place the food where they can handle it safely. If the pretzel stick was placed at position E, this child may have the same reaction that was described in Example #2 at the start of this chapter. An inability to lateralize the food to the molar ridge could result in gagging and vomiting. In contrast, placement of the pretzel stick at position A helps surpass the child's inability to lateralize the food and creates a more positive experience with it.

In many cases, children with neuromotor issues are being fed with their heads in extension. Put your head back and attempt to swallow. It is uncomfortable even if you have normal muscle tone. For clients with decreased postural stability and muscle tone issues, their airways are compromised every time they eat in this position. A therapeutic feeding program should include positioning to support postural stability.

Other factors in a therapeutic feeding program include: sensory-based food choices, utensils that support feeding skills, and techniques that support safe, effective eating. These specific techniques will be discussed in Chapter 9.

What is the ultimate goal of a feeding program?

Most children go through stages of "picky eating," and many people have food preferences secondary to cultural experiences and sensory-motor abilities. Some people have adequate nutrition, but they go through life as "picky eaters." Some clients' diets may be limited by medical, sensory, or neuromotor skills. Not every client in therapy will be an oral feeder. This book is intended for those individuals who have sensory-motor deficits that impact their ability to engage in safe-nutritive feedings.

The ultimate goals of a feeding program are:

1. **To ensure adequate nutrition.** If your client's medical concerns or sensory-motor systems cannot support oral feeding, then enteral (tube) feeding may be necessary to support brain growth and development.

2. **To ensure that the client has the sensory-motor skills to support safe, effective, nutritive feeding.**

This is not to say that behavioral issues do not develop. These issues will be addressed in Chapter 10; however, the etiology of food refusal is rarely behavioral and usually has sensory-motor underpinnings (Overland, 2011). Behavioral issues may need to be addressed; however, you will be much more effective in implementing a behavioral program if you first address the underlying sensory-motor issues.

CONCLUSION:

A sensory-motor approach encompasses sensory processing and oral sensory-motor skill development needed for safe, effective, nutritive feeding. This text will discuss: the oral phase of feeding, the factors that influence feeding, nutritional concerns, sensory-processing disorders, assessment, pre-feeding activities, sensory-based diet shaping, therapeutic feeding, and writing a program plan. It will also provide helpful forms and a cookbook to assist therapists who are treating children with oral sensory-motor feeding disorders.

CHAPTER 2:
THE ORAL PHASE OF FEEDING

LEADING GOALS/POINTS

Defining the Oral Phase of Feeding

Understanding key terminology of this text

Learning the Oral Sensory-Motor/Feeding Developmental Sequence

An overview of the Three Part Treatment Approach to Feeding and Speech Clarity

Defining the Oral Phase of Feeding

Feeding begins long before food enters the mouth. If a child sees or smells food and has a negative reaction, the feeding paradigm has begun. It is impossible to do feeding therapy without considering the whole child. The first step in understanding the intent of this text is to define the stages of feeding and swallowing. There are three phases of feeding: oral sensory-motor, pharyngeal, and esophageal (Arvedson & Bodsky, 2001). While these three phases can be described individually, they are all related.

FEEDING PARADIGM

FEEDING IS A TEAM APPROACH

In order to properly treat feeding disorders, you need to look at the client's medical status, sensory processing, motor development, the family paradigm, and caregiver-child connection during feeding. Feeding therapy is a team approach. Professionals who collaborate on this team could include: a speech-language pathologist, occupational therapist, physical therapist, internist, respiratory specialist, nutritionist, gastroenterologist, otolaryngologist, psychologist, and others as appropriate.

There are many valuable texts that focus on feeding in the NICU, breast and bottle feeding, and dysphagia (e.g., Ardveson & Brodsky, 2001). This text will be specifically on the oral phase of feeding.

The oral phase of feeding includes the following 3 stages:

1. Optimal level of arousal to allow the child to be organized for adequate feeding;

2. Sensory-motor development to support body positioning for feeding;

3. Oral sensory-motor skills to support the intake and management of food in preparation for swallowing.

In order to assess and treat children with oral phase feeding disorders, it is essential to understand key terms and the chronological development of oral sensory-motor skills necessary for feeding.

Key terms to be discussed in this text are defined as follows:

Bolus: The organization of food or medicine into a mass in the oral cavity.

Dissociation: The separation of movement, in order to complete a controlled task, which is secondary to stability.

Extension: Straightening or increasing the joint angle.

Feedback: Motor control processing in which sensory feedback is used for ongoing production of a skilled movement.

Feedforward: Anticipatory sensory information used to prepare for or initiate postural and movement requirements of a motor task.

Fixing: An abnormal posture used to compensate for reduced stability, dissociation, and/or grading.

Flexion: Decreasing or bending the joint angle.

Grading: Appropriately matching movement to the controlled task.

Hard-Wired Synergy: Patterns that develop in utero and are present at birth. These patterns are gradually inhibited by higher brain centers post natal.

Infant Reflexes: A hard-wired synergy present at birth. The emergence of reflexes and the age at which they disappear can be signs of neurological impairment. Reflexes are reactions to stimuli, and they indicate developmental maturation (Bahr 2001).

Kinesthetic System: The part of the sensory system that monitors movement of the body's muscles, tendons, and joints.

Lateral Reflex: A hard-wired synergy that is stimulated by stroking the lateral margin of the tongue which results in lateralization toward that stimulus.

Mastication: The process of chewing in which food is broken down.

Myofascial: Pertaining to or involving the fascia surrounding and associated with muscle tissue.

Phasic Bite: A hard-wired synergy/reflex in which an infant bites down in response to any object being placed intra-orally to protect the airway.

Postural Control: Control of the body's position in space for the purposes of maintaining the body's stability against the force of gravity and orientation of the body's segments to each other in task-specific relationships (Shumway-Cook & Woollacott 2001; Bahr 2001).

Postural Tone: The distribution of muscle tone among anti-gravity muscles that are constrained to act together to maintain posture against the force of gravity and simultaneously adapt stiffness to allow the flexibility necessary for movement (Shumway-Cook and Woollacott 2001).

Proprioception: The sense of the orientation of one's limbs in space.

Rooting: A reflex that is seen in normal newborn babies, who automatically turn the face toward the stimulus, and make sucking motions with the mouth when the cheek or lip is touched. The rooting reflex helps to ensure successful breastfeeding.

Sensory Integration: The neurological process that organizes sensation from one's own body and the environment, thus making it possible to use the body effectively within the environment.

Sensory Processing: Related to the observed behavior when an individual has difficulty taking information in from the environment, and acting on it appropriately.

Stability: The ability to maintain the center of mass over the base of support.

Suck: A suck is a sequence of reflexes and sensory-motor planning that allows a newborn to feed from a breast or bottle. An infant orients to the nipple (rooting response), opens the mouth widely (gape response), brings the tongue down to the floor of the mouth, extends it over the lower lip to grasp the nipple. The mouth closes, the anterior tongue cups to hold the nipple, the body of the tongue grooves to stabilize the nipple. The nipple is enclosed between the grooved tongue, cheeks, and palate, forming a teat. The nipple should contact the infant's posterior hard palate. After attachment, the infant holds the nipple with the anterior and mid-tongue with the lips assisting, the soft palate hinges downward contacting the back of the tongue, the nipple is sealed between soft palate, grooved tongue, lips, and cheeks. The tongue is grooved from front to back, milk sprays from the nipple and forms a bolus, the soft palate elevates, pharyngeal walls contract (to close off the nasal passage), vocal folds are closed by arytenoid cartilage moving together. The epiglottis tilts down to direct milk around vocal folds, suprahyoid muscles pull the larynx upward to shorten the pharynx, and the tongue uses positive pressure to push the bolus of milk into the pharynx for transit to the esophagus (Genna, 2012).

Sucking: This refers to the oral motor activity that transfers milk during breast (or bottle) feeding. Electromyogram (EMG) studies by Geddes, Kent and Hartmann in 2008, showed that sucking does not change from reflexive to active in breast-fed infants. Sucking may change from passive to active in bottle-fed infants (C.W. Genna, personal communication, July 20, 2012).

Suckling: This refers to the act of feeding at the breast (Genna, 2012).

Suckle: This refers to an abnormal movement in breast/bottle feeding when the infant using a back and forth movement of the tongue, which is never typical (Genna, 2012).

NOTE: Older literature proposes that suckling is an in/out movement of the tongue, which becomes more active or a "true suck", at around three months of age (Morris & Klein, 1987). According to recent studies by lactation specialists, this may be due to the mechanical differences between breast and bottle feeding, or growth of the oral cavity in comparison to the relationship of the static artificial nipple. Therefore, there may be a change in motor skills for bottle feeding, but not for the breast (C.W. Genna, personal communication, July 20, 2012).

Tactile: The sense of touch.

Tone: The amount of contraction in a muscle.

Vestibular System: The part of the sensory system that contributes to balance and movement. It is regulated by the cochlea, and the labyrinth of the inner ear.

Oral Sensory-Motor/Feeding Development Sequence

In order to evaluate atypical or compensatory feeding skills, it is important to know the typical developmental sequence of oral motor skills for feeding.

0-3 months
- Rooting reflex
- Suck reflex
- Suck-swallow reflex
- Phasic bite reflex
- Lateral tongue reflex
- Gag reflex on front third of tongue
- Tongue cups to provide channel for backward movement of liquid
- Fatty sucking pads, lips, tongue, and palate function as a unit

The newborn baby's first job is to self-regulate for feeding. Newborns are driven by hard-wired synergies or reflexes. The rooting reflex is stimulated with touch to the cheeks or lips. This allows the infant to find the breast or bottle. In a full-term infant (i.e. born at 40 weeks gestation), a suck is stimulated with touch to the lips or tongue. There is a 1:1 correspondence between a suck and a swallow in a full-term newborn (Genna, 2012). At this point the suck is non-dissociated, meaning the lips, tongue, jaw, and fatty sucking pads are all working together. The suck, swallow, breathe synchrony describes the coordination of the systems for feeding. The soft cupping of the tongue allows the infant to channel the liquid. The phasic bite reflex is stimulated with input to the lateral molar ridge. The infant will "munch" (open and close the jaw), in response to the stimulus. Stimulation to the lateral border of the tongue will result in movement of the tongue laterally to the input. At birth, the gag reflex is on the front third of the tongue. Infants are hard-wired with skills that allow them to successfully breast or bottle feed.

INFANTS ARE BORN WITH HARD-WIRED SYNERGIES

4-6 Months
- Rooting reflex comes under control between 4-6 months
- Phasic bite comes under control by five months
- Munch chew pattern is active between 5-6 months
- Decreased coordination of suck, swallow, breathe as the suck becomes more active
- Gag reflex is moving back/slightly less sensitive
- Protrusion/retraction of the tongue in anticipation of the spoon
- Protrusion/retraction to swallow food/liquid

In the 4-6 month period, the infant is coming out of physiological flexion. Oral motor skills are becoming more active and volitional rather than reflexive. At this point the aforementioned rooting reflex is being integrated, while an active munch chew pattern replaces the phasic bite. As the suck becomes more active there may be decreased coordination of the suck, swallow, breathe synchrony. Spoon-feeding is often introduced at around six months, but protrusion/retraction of the tongue may persist in anticipation of the spoon. The gag reflex is moving back, allowing for the infant to tolerate spoon-feeding.

7-9 months
- Lateral tongue reflex comes under control by 6-8 months
- Mixed tongue movements in/out, up/down, side to side
- Active lip movements; some jaw/lip dissociation for spoon-feeding, lip closure for swallowing purees
- Cup drinking—jaw is still unstable
- Some protrusion/retraction to facilitate a swallow persists
- Munch chew with food placed on lateral molar ridge (rhythmic bite)
- Beginning of active transfer of food from side to center, center to side
- Some diagonal/rotary jaw movement
- Gag reflex is on back third of tongue
- Teething begins between 5-9 months

Reflexive movements continue to become integrated motor skills. The lateral tongue reflex comes under control, and active tongue lateralization to move a solid bolus is emerging. Active lip movement to clear a pureed bolus from a spoon should be emerging. A rhythmic bite, or munch chew, can be observed with the introduction of solid foods, such as a Gerber Puff®. Tongue movement can be observed to move food from the middle of the mouth, to the side of the mouth, and back to the middle. At this point, tongue protrusion is still observed to facilitate a swallow. The gag reflex has moved to the back third of the tongue allowing the infant to explore solid foods.

10-12 months

- True suck is well established
- Improved lip closure for swallowing liquids
- Cleans lower lip with teeth
- Upper lip moves down and forward and lower lip moves in to remove a pureed bolus from a spoon
- Improved coordination during drinking
- Rotary chew pattern is developing
- Active lip, cheek movement during chewing
- Gag reflex moves back towards the pharyngeal wall

This is an important time period for the introduction of solid foods. A rotary chew pattern is developing, and babies have the ability to handle a variety of food textures. Dissociated lip mobility is observed for spoon feeding. Straw drinking can be introduced and is effective for nutrition.

13-15 months

- Developing jaw, lip, tongue dissociation
- Dissociation of tongue blade and tongue tip
- Increased dynamic jaw stability for biting
- Some lip closure during chewing
- Can maintain a continuous suck during cup drinking

The toddler is beginning to use the tongue tip and the lateral borders of the tongue to move food to the molar ridge for chewing. As jaw stability improves, emerging dissociation of jaw, lips, and tongue can be observed.

16-18 months
- Good internal jaw stability is developing
- Increased dissociation of jaw/lip/tongue movement
- Reduced tongue protrusion to support swallowing
- Good control of liquid
- Controlled bite (i.e., Cookie or pretzel) without associated head movement
- Smoother integration of tongue, lip and jaw movements

Typically developing toddlers are enjoying family foods at this point.

19-24 months
- Uses tongue to clean lips
- Can straw drink (suck with long sequences)
- Can chew with lips closed
- Tongue retraction for swallowing
- Chews meats completely
- Rotary chew

A rotary chew pattern can be observed with most food textures. The toddler should have tongue retraction for swallowing most solid foods and liquids.

25-36 months
- Internal jaw stabilization
- Tongue tip elevation for swallowing
- Appropriate jaw grading for biting and chewing
- Gradual refinement of tongue movements
- Circular rotary chew patterns ("adult" pattern)
- Mature swallow pattern

By 36 months of age, a child has an "adult-like" motor plan for feeding. Strength and stability continue to develop. Tongue thrusting to support swallowing is resolved.

The Three-Part Approach to Feeding and Speech Development

Since we have discussed the early developing stages of oral sensory-motor development, it seems appropriate to discuss the interaction between this development and speech.

Children with oral sensory-motor feeding disorders often have concurrent speech clarity issues. The Three-Part Treatment Approach addresses oral sensory-motor skills to support feeding, and Oral Placement skills to support sound production. Oral Placement is a term coined by Sara Rosenfeld Johnson and Diane Bahr in 2010 (Bahr & Rosenfeld-Johnson, 2010). Oral Placement Therapy (OPT) is used when a client cannot produce the standard speech sound using traditional approaches that rely on "Look at me, listen to me, and say what I say." OPT adds the tactile component or the "feel" of speech. TalkTools® unique therapy tools are used to teach articulator awareness, placement, and muscle memory (Moore & Ruark, 1996). Once the client is able to produce the required placement, the speech sound is immediately introduced along with traditional interventions (Bahr & Johnson, 2010). Therefore, it is important to understand while the research is still emerging to support the correlation between oral placement and speech production, that using oral tactile techniques for speech is not a new concept. The use of "tools" in speech therapy dates back to 1939 (Marshalla, 2012).

The correlation between oral sensory-motor skills and feeding has already been supported by evidenced based practice, and will be cited throughout this text. The body is a dynamic system. While there is not a 1:1 correspondence between the oral sensory-motor skills for feeding and the oral sensory-motor skills for speech, there is an overlay of one system to another. Feeding and speech production are discreet processes with discreet motor plans. The focus of this book is the oral

THE BODY IS A DYNAMIC SYSTEM

phase of feeding; however, it should be noted that the underlying motor skills to support speech are also being targeted. This is the foundation of the Three-Part Treatment Approach. This text can be used in conjunction with Sara Rosenfeld-Johnson's *Oral Placement Therapy for Speech and Feeding*.

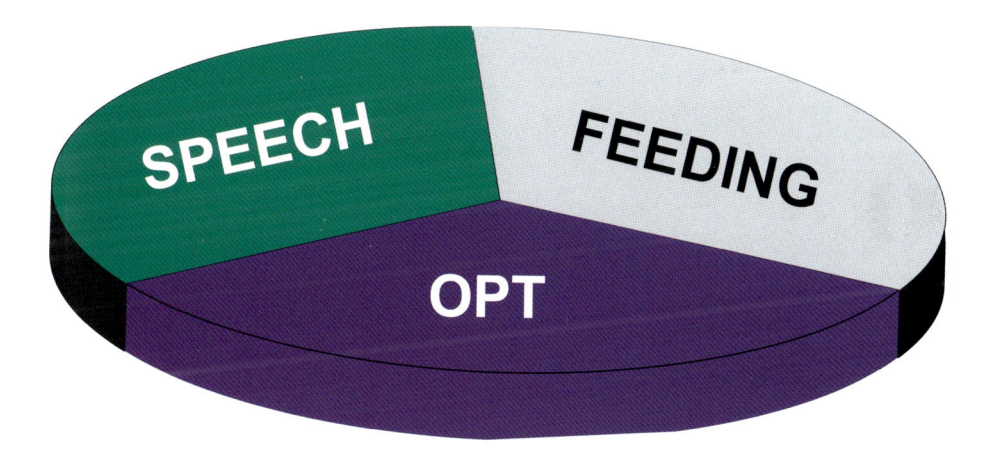

CONCLUSION:

In order to diagnose and treat oral sensory-motor feeding disorders, we must understand typical development. This chapter has outlined the hard-wired synergies and motor skill sets that develop in the first three years of life. These oral sensory-motor skills are important for feeding. While there is not a 1:1 ratio for speech production, there is certainly a correlation; therefore pre-feeding activities are a very important part of the TalkTools® Three-Part Treatment Approach for speech clarity and feeding.

CHAPTER 3:
FACTORS THAT INFLUENCE FEEDING

LEADING GOALS/POINTS

Understanding muscle tone

Recognizing structural anomalies

Understanding how medical issues impact the oral phase of feeding

The purpose of this chapter is to discuss the multiple factors that influence the oral phase of feeding that may include but are not limited to: muscle tone, structure, metabolic issues, prematurity, respiratory and cardiac issues, and reflux. The oral phase of feeding includes: intake of food into the oral cavity, preparation/management of the bolus, and oral transport/transit in preparation for swallowing. Infants are born with hard-wired synergies, or reflexes, that support the oral phase of feeding. These synergies mature into volitional sensory-motor skills secondary to the infant's experiences with the environment and feeding. It is important to know the typical development of sensory-motor skills that support feeding. This topic was discussed in Chapter 2 of this text. Any breakdown in oral motor skill development can result in compensatory feeding strategies, sensory issues, and/or food refusal.

Muscle Tone

Muscle tone is the natural tension of a muscle at rest. It is the continuous, passive, and partial contraction of the muscles, or the muscle's resistance to passive stretch during a resting state. It helps maintain posture.

Unconscious nerve impulses maintain the muscles in a partially contracted state. If a sudden pull or stretch occurs, the body responds by automatically increasing the muscle's tension, a reflex that helps guard against danger, as well as helps to maintain balance.

Tone has a "default" or "steady state." There is, for the most part, no actual "rest state" because the nerves are constantly firing to maintain a rest posture. Both the extensor (serves to straighten) and flexor (serves to bend), under normal intervention, maintain constant muscle tone while "at rest," and this maintains "normal" posture (Morris & Klein, 2000).

Physical disorders can result in abnormally low (hypotonia) or high (hypertonia) muscle tone. This impacts not only movement but the "rest state" or "normal" posture.

Hypotonia is not a specific medical disorder, but a potential symptom of many different diseases and disorders that affect motor nerve function beginning in the brain as muscle strength.

Recognizing hypotonia, even in early infancy, is usually relatively straightforward to the trained eye, but diagnosing the underlying cause of the hypotonia can be challenging at times. While it is rarely available for clinicians, instrumental testing for muscle tone would be preferred. The long-term effects of hypotonia on a child's development and later life depend primarily on the severity of the resulting muscle weakness and the cause.

FLACCIDITY

Hypotonia usually presents as muscle flaccidity (lax ligaments) where the limbs appear floppy, stretch reflex responses are decreased, and the limb's resistance to passive movement is also decreased. Many individuals with hypotonia eventually have mixed muscle tone due to compensatory fixing patterns used (Bahr, 2001).

Hypotonia is seen in many genetic and developmental disabilities, including but not limited to:

- Prader-Willi syndrome
- Williams syndrome
- Trisomy 21, or Down syndrome

- Marfan syndrome
- Muscular Dystrophy
- Mitochondrial disorders
- Meningitis
- Encephalitis
- Guillain-Barre syndrome
- Congenital hypothyroidism
- Hypotonic cerebral palsy
- Benign congenital hypotonia

RIGIDITY

Hypertonia is a condition marked by an atypical increase in muscle tension and an inability for the muscle to stretch, that results from injury, disease, or medical conditions. It is caused by injury to motor pathways in the central nervous system that carry information from the central nervous system to the muscles that control posture, muscle tone, and reflexes. It is seen in upper motor neuron diseases where there are lesions in the pyramidal tract and extrapyramidal tract. In its most severe form, hypertonia can result in deformity of the muscles and joints.

Hypertonia can present clinically as rigidity. It is differentiated from spasticity. Rigidity is an involuntary stiffening or straightening out of muscles, accompanied by abnormally increased muscle tone and the reduced ability of a muscle to stretch. This type of hypertonia is most common in Parkinson's Disease.

Spasticity involves uncontrollable muscle spasms, stiffening or straightening out of muscles, shock-like **SPASTICITY** contractions of all or part of a group of muscles, and abnormal muscle tone. It is seen in disorders such as cerebral palsy, stroke, and spinal cord injury.

Dystonic hypertonia refers to muscle resistance during passive stretching, and a tendency of a limb to return to a fixed involuntary (and sometimes abnormal) posture following movement.

Therapeutically, it is important to understand muscle tone. Muscle tone cannot be changed; however, therapists can work to improve graded strength and dissociation of movement in muscle groups, which may lead to improved sensory-motor pathways for muscle function. The National Institute of Neurological Disorders and Stroke stated that physical therapy can improve motor control and overall body strength in individuals with hypotonia (NIDS, 2008). This is crucial for maintaining both static and dynamic postural stability, which is important since postural instability is a common problem in people with hypotonia. Physical therapists might use sensory/neuromuscular stimulation techniques such as: quick stretch, resistance, or tapping to enhance muscle contraction in patients with hypotonia. For patients who demonstrate muscle weakness secondary to hypotonia, strengthening exercises that do not overload the muscles but help to develop graded strength are indicated.

These principles of physical therapy are important to note when dealing with individuals who present with oral-facial hypotonia. Reduced tone of the jaw, lip, cheeks, and tongue may result in disorders of mastication, speech, and swallowing. Oral-facial hypotonia is related to feeding disorders as it impacts the pre-feeding skills necessary to manage a bolus and prepare it for the swallow. When working on feeding skills, the therapist should follow the same principles of maintaining postural stability. What is seen in the body will also be seen in the mouth.

Hypertonia can also negatively impact feeding skills due to a lack of motor control. Therapy tasks often involve relaxation of the muscles, as well as targeting mobility and stability. Hypertonia and fixing are just as problematic and require interventions.

Structure

The cranio-facial structure is a complex one. Neurology and anatomy texts describe in detail the complex system of

CRANIOFACIAL STRUCTURES

muscles and nerves of the face, mouth, head, and neck. We will be discussing these structures as they relate to feeding skills.

At birth, head circumference is always measured. A small head circumference can mean several things:

1) Genetics play a role in the size of the head.

2) An infant may tend to have smaller than average head size.

3) The head measurements may simply reflect his or her genetic heritage. However, it may also mean that the baby's brain is not growing well. This is called microcephaly, which may result in limited brain development.

A large head circumference can also be clinically significant. As with small head sizes, genetics can also play a role in large head sizes. A large head size may signal hydrocephalus, resulting from an excessive amount of fluid in the brain's ventricles and tissues surrounding the brain. This results in compression of the normal brain tissue and impairs the brain's neurological function and growth.

It is important to note in a case history if microcephaly or hydrocephalus was present at birth because of the developmental disabilities that may be associated with these conditions.

While the size and, sometimes, shape of the head is important, the symmetry of the face itself is important to analyze in an assessment. The head is divided into sections based on vertical and horizontal planes. This is the Facial Index Analysis (Boshart, 2001; Boshart, 1999; Bahr, 2010).

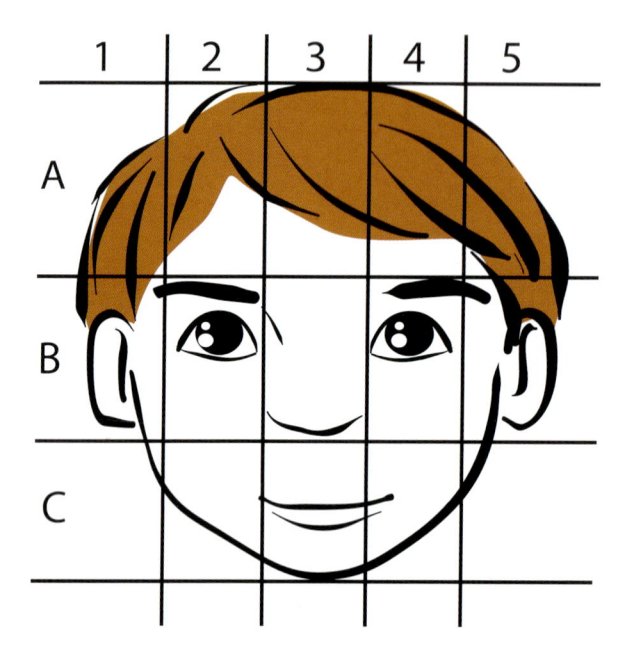

Vertical: Equal Thirds A-B-C
Horizontal: Equal Fifths 1-2-3-4-5

An individual with equal horizontal widths is considered typical or mesocephalic. An individual with narrow widths, especially in areas 2, 3, or 4 are considered to have narrow facial angles, which are called dolicocephalic. A person with wide angles especially in 1, 3, and 5 is considered to be brachyecephalic (Boshart, 2001; Boshart, 1999).

It is important when analyzing the oral-facial structures to look for excessive bone growth or asymmetry in the face. It is also important to compare the shape of the palate with facial angles. A narrow high palate in a dolicocephalic structure is common, whereas a narrow high palate in a mesocephalic or bracheycephalic structure would indicate a deviation in intraoral tongue resting posture (Merkel-Walsh, 2012).

Asymmetry, or malocclusion of the maxilla and mandible, causes skewing and displacement of the tongue, which leads to malformation of the hard palate. A high palatal vault increases tongue to palate distance, making the intraoral seal for swallowing challenging. A wide vault in the palate may interfere with stabilization for the tongue. Narrowing of the front of the palate often causes the tongue to protrude or retract excessively.

The Facial Index also includes analysis of the profile of the face. This is directly related to dental alignment. Diagram A shows a normal molar occlusion (Angle's Class I) with a normal profile. Diagram B shows a distoclusion (Angle's Class II), and a convex facial profile (Merkel, 2002). This is often seen in individuals with myofunctional disorders and macrognosia. Diagram C shows a mesioclusion (Angle's Class III), and a convex facial structure often associated with an underbite, and myofunctional issues. It is important to understand that Angle's classification system is the description of the molar alignment and not the incisor alignment (Merkel-Walsh, 2001). If the dentition is not in alignment, this could impact mastication or lip closure, both of which are important for chewing and bolus preparation (Merkel-Walsh, 2001).

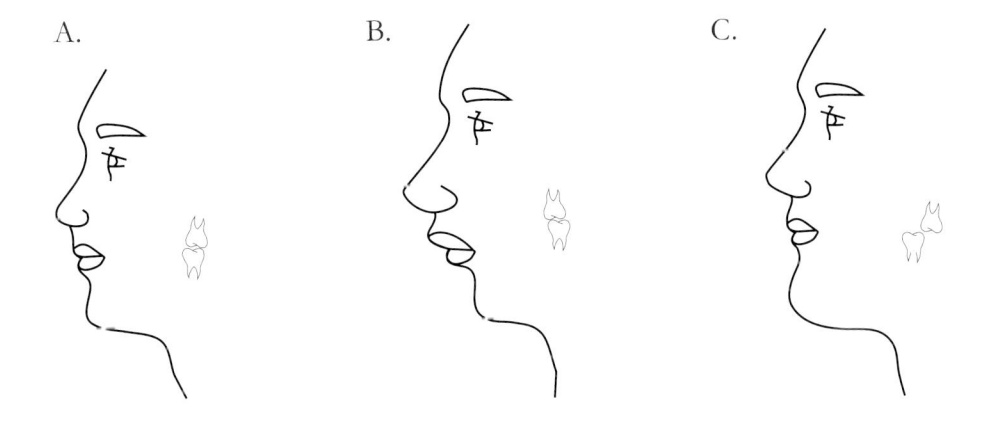

A. B. C.

When there are Class II or Class III maloclussions, there are almost always lingual issues. In addition, functional malocclusions of the central dentition (eye teeth and central incisors) are often associated.

Note: The following diagrams show the sagital (side) view of the relationship between the upper central incisor to the lower central incisor (Merkel-Walsh, 2002).

Open Bite: The client presents with normal molar alignment (Class I); however, there is no contact between the central incisors (the two upper and lower teeth at the mouth midline).

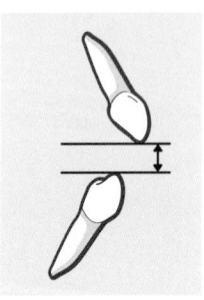

Overjet: Similar to the open bite, there is no contact between the central incisors; however, in this case, the top teeth have a horizontal projection.

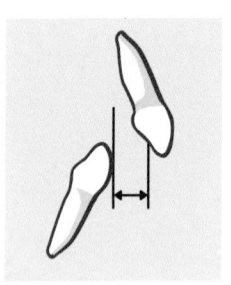

Overbite or Underbite: The molar alignment is normal; however, the relationship of the central incisors is not normal. In an overbite, the maxillary incisors overlap the mandibular incisors. In an underbite, the mandibular incisors overlap the maxillary incisors.

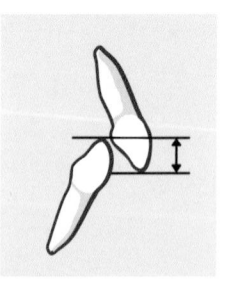

Typically individuals with Class II Distoclusion also present with an open bite or overjet, and individuals with Class III Mesioclusion often present with an underbite; however any combination of symptoms can occur, so it is critical to analyze the dentition carefully. Finally, some individuals can present with a crossbite, in which the left molar alignment differs from the right. For example the child has Class I on the right, and Class III on the left.

The use of appropriately chosen and systematically applied oral sensory-motor techniques can positively impact cranio-facial development (Pierce, 1980). Infants who are predisposed to these conditions from genetic and chromosomal imbalances, such as Down syndrome, are at risk and should be treated proactively at birth.

Structural differences are frequently found in individuals who have abnormalities of the soft tissue. This occurs because the muscles are not working properly to facilitate structural alignment, particularly once the child is upright and against the force of gravity. This includes but is not limited to:

- Charge Syndrome
- Cleft Lip
- Cleft Palate
- Crouzon Syndrome
- Facial Palsy
- Frontonasal Dyplasia
- Goldenhar Syndrome
- Microtia
- Miller Syndrome
- Moebius Syndrome
- Pierre Robin Syndrome
- Treacher Collins Syndrome
- Velocardial Facial Syndrome

Another common structural deviation that significantly impacts feeding is a restrictive sublingual frenum and/or restricted labial frenums (Hanson & Mason, 2003).

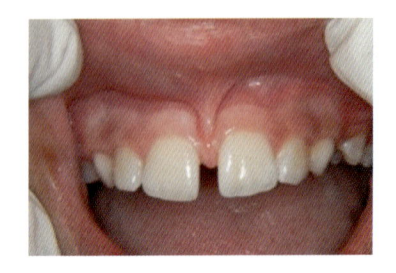

The Labial Frenum is a little tag of tissue in the center of the upper and the lower lip that attaches the lip to the gums. It is not especially useful, and sometimes causes orthodontic or periodontal problems if the attachment on the gums is too close to the teeth. On a cosmetic level, it can cause a space in between the two top central incisors. On a functional level, it can lead to poor lip movement during spoon feeding or bilabial speech sound production, and subsequent upper lip insufficiency (Boshart, 1999). If it is too thick, or restrictive, it can be shaved down or removed. The procedure is called a frenectomy. This is most often performed by an oral surgeon.

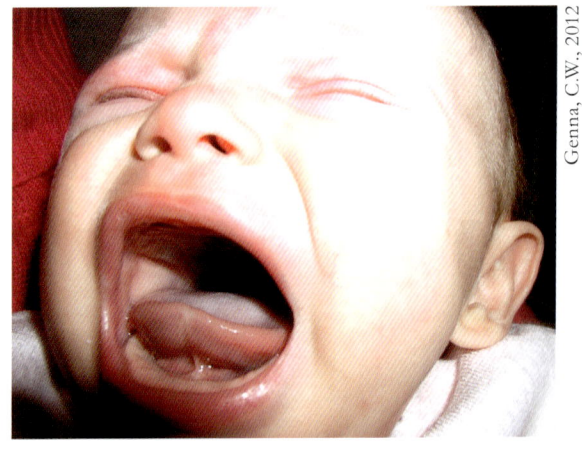

The thin strip of tissue that runs vertically from the floor of the mouth to the undersurface of the tongue is called the lingual frenum. If it is too short, too close to the tongue tip, or too taut, it can limit movement of the tongue, specifically retraction, lateralization, and elevation (Palmer, 2001). If the frenum is attached too far back, this is a posterior tongue tie, which pulls the midsection of the tongue down and restricts lateral movement. In some cases, it is so short that it actually interferes with feeding, oral hygiene, and speaking. This is sometimes noted immediately at birth because it interferes with breast and/or bottle feeding. If the lingual frenum is restricted, it can be clipped with surgical scissors or a laser. The procedure is called a lingual frenectomy. This is most often performed by an oral surgeon or an otolaryngologist (ENT).

Metabolic Issues

Metabolism is the process the body uses to get or make energy from food. Food is made up of proteins, carbohydrates, and fats. Chemicals in the digestive system break the food parts down into sugars and acids, which is essentially the body's fuel. The body can use this fuel right away, or it can store the energy in body tissue, muscles, and fat.

A metabolic disorder occurs when abnormal chemical reactions in the body disrupt this process. When this happens, there can be an imbalance of hormones, sugars, and fats that need to stay regulated in order to maintain a healthy body.

THE PROCESS OF BREAKING DOWN FOODS

Metabolic disorders include but are not limited to:

- Barth Syndrome
- Cystic Fibrosis
- Diabetes
- Diseases of the thyroid
- Hypoglycemia
- Inborn error of metabolism
- Lactose Intolerance
- Polycystic Ovaries
- Ricket's Disease
- Sanfillipo Syndrome

When an individual with a feeding disorder has co-existing metabolic issues, it is imperative to consult and work with the treating physician and dietitian, in terms of target foods and caloric intake, to ensure absorption of calories, fats, and sugars.

Prematurity

Most pregnancies last around 40 weeks. Babies born between 37 and 39 weeks are called near term. Babies between 40 and 42 completed weeks of pregnancy are called full term. According to the American Pregnancy Association, a baby born before 37 weeks' gestation is considered premature (premie).

Medical factors may contribute to prematurity, but in some cases, the cause of prematurity is unknown. The earlier a baby is born, the more likely he/she is to have complications. Complications in premature newborns are managed in the Neonatal Intensive Care Unit (NICU).

The most common complications of prematurity are: immature lung function, jaundice, feeding difficulties, and infection. Heart and digestive complications may also be present. According to the March of Dimes, serious infections in premature babies include sepsis (which is a blood infection), pneumonia, and meningitis (an infection of the membranes surrounding the brain). To help protect premature babies from infection, they are placed in incubators in a NICU (March of Dimes, 2012). The use of an incubator also helps to maintain a warm environment for the baby. Because premature babies have little or no body fat, or fatty sucking pads, they also have difficulty maintaining an adequate temperature outside of the womb (Bahr, 2010).

The time the infant spends in the NICU depends on when they were born, the complexity of the delivery and the development of the organs. Feeding skills play a large part in determining when a newborn can leave a NICU.

Feeding complications in preemies often involve problems with the development of the suck–swallow-breathe reflex that allows a newborn to suck a nipple. This is a hard-wired synergy that develops between 32-34 weeks of gestation. When the baby is born prematurely, he/she often has not developed this innate skill in the womb, and therefore must be tube fed until the skill is developed and the infant can participate in oral feedings.

Some common feeding issues in premies are:

1. **Hypoxemia:** This is a loss of oxygen during oral feedings. Additional oxygen may be needed at the time of feedings, or the infant may need breaks to reduce respiratory fatigue.

2. **Fatigue:** The premie does not have the muscle stamina to support a full feed, and therefore may fall asleep.

3. **Sensory processing issues:** A hospital can be noisy, have bright lights, and be overwhelming for the premie.

4. **Satiation levels:** Premies can usually only handle small amounts of breast milk or formula at feedings, and may need to be given concentrated calories.

5. **Respiration issues:** The ability to suck and swallow is developed in utero; however, the suck-swallow-breathe reflex is underdeveloped, and therefore, feedings may cause lung fatigue. Respiratory Distress Syndrome (RDS) is common in premies.

6. **Decreased hunger:** Because the infant was born before its due date, they often do not experience hunger until it is closer to their true birth date.

7. **Digestive issues:** Gastroesophogeal Reflux Disease (GERD) and Necrotizing enterocolitis (NEC) are common in premies, and both can impact oral feeding and nutritional absorption.

Respiratory and Cardiac Issues

As aforementioned in the discussion of premature birth, respiratory and/or cardiac issues can have an impact on feedings. Diseases of the lung and/or heart can exist at any age. In fact, cardiac and respiratory diseases are often concurrent.

Broncopulmonary Dysplasia (BPD) is a common issue seen in a variety of developmental disabilities, especially in premies and children with low birth weight. Infants and young children with severe BPD may require ongoing mechanical ventilation and tracheotomy. They may also have great nutritional concerns. Corticosteroids, diuretics, and gastrostomy tube feedings may all affect growth and nutrition. Feeding problems are common in infants with moderate to severe BPD. Problems found in infants with BPD include poor coordination of sucking, swallowing, and breathing; swallowing dysfunction with silent microaspiration; oral-tactile hypersensitivity; and gastroesophageal reflux; and/or delayed gastric emptying. Asthma is another chronic respiratory disease that affects the airways and should be considered in feeding therapy.

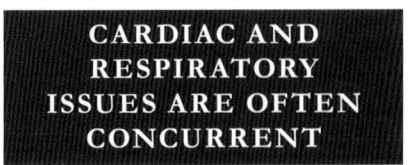

> **CARDIAC AND RESPIRATORY ISSUES ARE OFTEN CONCURRENT**

Cardiac issues can be very complex in dealing with feeding disorders. Symptoms of heart attack and dysphagia (difficulty swallowing) can often mimic one another in adult patients. Feeding issues often follow a heart attack, and respiratory fatigue during feedings can cause rapid heart rate and coronary distress.

Reflux

Gastroesophageal reflux disease (GERD), also called gastro-oesophageal reflux disease (GORD), gastric reflux disease, or acid reflux disease is often chronic, resulting in mucosal damage caused by stomach acid coming up from the stomach into the esophagus. The typical symptom is called "heartburn."

GERD is usually caused by changes in the barrier between the stomach and the esophagus, including abnormal relaxation of the lower esophageal sphincter, which normally holds the top of the stomach closed; impaired expulsion of gastric reflux from the esophagus; or a hiatal hernia.

GERD is especially common in clients who are premature, have muscle tone issues, or food allergies. There is an improving awareness in the medical community of diagnosing GERD in infants.

Symptoms of GERD in infancy include:

- Irritability during feedings
- Sleep issues
- Food refusal
- Chronic vomiting
- Pulling the knees into the chest
- "Colic"
- Wet burps
- Frequent coughing
- Hoarseness
- Wheezing
- Chronic hiccups
- Sour breath

Treatment for GERD traditionally involves medication (such as Pepcid®, Mylanta® or Prevacid®); however, there is limited research supporting the efficacy of reflux medication in the premature infant population.

Other treatments involve changes in diet; for example, changing an infant's formula if there are food sensitivities or intolerances. Several prescription formulas can be utilized, such as Neocate®, that are free of soy and dairy. In less severe cases, over-the-counter predigested formulas are available such as: Gentlease® and Alimentum®. For those babies who are breast fed, the mother may be asked to limit her diet to restrict trigger foods such as dairy and soy. Natural remedies such as gripe water and probiotics are increasingly popular and available over the counter.

Pre-thickened formulas such as Enfamil AR®, commercial thickeners like Simply Thick® and rice cereal were traditionally used to help with GERD. While rice cereal may be necessary for infants who aspirate, there is debate in the literature about whether any thickeners should be used with infants (Huang et al., 2002). Rice cereal may decrease motility that is already compromised in premature infants and infants with tone issues. Some thickeners have been correlated with increased incidences of NEC (Shrader & Associates, 2011).

Bottle selection is very important when feeding an infant with GERD. Dr. Brown's®, The Playtex Nurser® and Advent® are all popular BPA-free bottle systems. They prevent the infant from ingesting air, which further aggravates the reflux.

Infants with GERD need special accommodations in terms of size of the bolus and frequency of the feeds. In general it is best to concentrate feedings with decreased liquid, frequent burping, and less time between feedings. Large bolus feeds can cause vomiting and severe discomfort. In addition, the infant should be in an upright position for at least 30 minutes after a feeding. Quality belly-time on a wedged pillow is also helpful (Morris & Klein, 2000). Positioning of the infant has been found to be very helpful in management of infants with GERD. Many positioners are now available such as a Boppy® Pillow or a reflux wedge, to ensure that the infant's ears are always angled above the mouth during and after feedings. This prevents regurgitation during the feeds, and reflux from going into the ear canals.

CONCLUSION:

There are many factors that influence the oral phase of feeding and can impact oral sensory-motor functioning. While some factors are more obvious, such as: structural deficits and prematurity, other factors need careful consideration and can be more difficult to diagnose, such as reflux. Understanding these factors will be critical for assessment and program planning.

CHAPTER 4:
NUTRITIONAL CONCERNS

LEADING GOALS/POINTS

Overview of basic nutrition

Understanding organic versus nonorganic Failure to Thrive (FTT)

Types of tube feedings

Understanding nutritional deficiencies

Awareness of specialized diets

Consideration of food allergies and intolerances

Food and drug interactions

On a feeding team, many specialists work together when dealing with nutritional concerns. Nutrition is how a living organism processes food for growth and for the replacement of tissues. The role of a nutritionist is to set forth guidelines for diet and weight maintenance. The physician, speech-language pathologist, occupational therapist, nutritionist, physical therapist, respiratory specialist, and family members all collaborate to determine diet management for optimal health.

This chapter will address nutritional concerns a feeding team may face when working with individuals who have various feeding disorders. While the nutritionist is responsible for assessing calories, calculating calories, and prescribing vitamins, diets, dietary and mineral supplements, it is helpful if the other therapists involved in this team possess a basic understanding of these topics, as they are all part of a collaborative model.

To better understand nutritional deficiency, it is helpful if we understand the dietary norms for children. Basic nutrition is as follows:

There are various types of nutritional deficits a feeding team may encounter. Examples are as follows:

MyPlate Suggested Calories & Intake Amounts for Children Ages 2 to 18 Years*

Food Group	Age 2-3 Years 1000-1400 Calories**	Age 4-8 Years 1200-2000 Calories**	Age 9-13 Years 1600-2600 Calories**	Age 14-18 Years 2000-3200 Calories**
Fruits	1 cup	1 cup to 1.5 cups	1.5 cups	2 cups
	Fresh, frozen, canned, dried fruit and fruit juices. 1 cup fruit or 100% juice or ½ cup dried fruit = 1 cup			
Vegetables	1 cup	1.5 cups	2 cups to 2.5 cups	2.5 cups to 3 cups
	Fresh, frozen, canned, dried vegetable and vegetable juices. Dark green, orange, legumes, starchy and other vegetables have specific recommendations[1]. 1 cup raw, cooked vegetable or vegetable juice or 2 cups raw leafy greens are considered 1 cup			
Grains	3 oz-eq	5 oz eq	5 oz eq to 6 oz eq	6 oz eq to 8 oz eq
	All foods made from rice, oats, barley, wheat, including bread, pasta, oatmeal, cereals, and crackers. 1 slice bread, 1 cup dry cereal, ½ cup cooked rice, cereal or pasta = 1 oz equivalent. Make half of all grains whole grains.			
Dairy	2 cups	2.5 cups	3 cups	3 cups
	All fluid milk and products made from milk. Does not include cream and butter. 1 cup milk or yogurt, 1.5 oz cheese, 2 oz processed cheese = 1 cup. 1 cup of soymilk counts as 1 cup in the Dairy Group.			
Protein Foods	2 oz eq	4 oz eq	5 oz eq	5 oz eq to 6.5 oz eq
	1 oz lean meat, fish, poultry, 1 egg, 1 Tbsp. peanut butter, ¼ cup cooked dry beans, ½ oz nuts/seeds = 1 oz eq			
Oils (Allowance per day)	3 tsp	4 tsp	5 tsp	5 tsp to 6 tsp
	Sources such as corn, safflower, sunflower, canola, corn, olive oils, as well as some nuts, fish, avocados, mayonnaise, salad dressings and margarine.			

*Recommendations will vary within stated ranges for males, females and ages. Please refer to www.MyPlate.gov for detailed recommendations.
**Based on activity levels of 'Sedentary' < 30 minutes per day, 'Mod. Active' 30-60 minutes per day, and 'Active' > 60 minutes per day, and calculations for Estimated Energy Requirements (EER) from the Institute of Medicine.
[1]Vegetable subgroup amounts per week can be found at www.MyPlate.gov.
Source: United States Department of Agriculture Center for Nutrition Policy and Promotion.

Provided by Cindy Baranoski MS, RD, LDN - Easter Seals DuPage & the Fox Valley Region

Failure to thrive

Failure to Thrive (FTT) is defined as a significant interruption in the expected rate of growth during early childhood. It is most often the first red flag in infancy that alerts the parent and/or pediatrician that there is a breakdown in the oral sensory-motor, feeding, and/or digestion system (Cole & Lanham, 2011). FTT can be the result of any breakdown in the nutritional chain that outlines the components of calories (the body's energy currency) and non-calories (the body's hydration, vitamins, and minerals). The body uses calories when it burns energy, and what it does not use is stored as fat. There is also a direct correlation between adequate nutrition and muscle tone (Dorfman, n.d.).

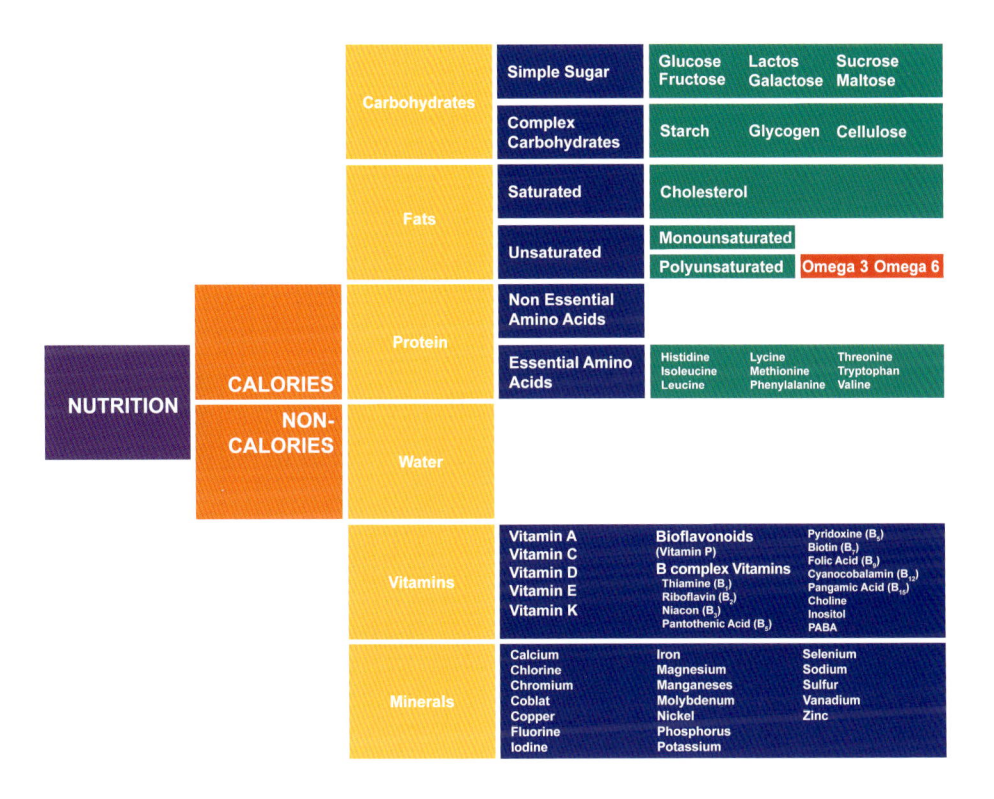

NUTRITION	CALORIES	Carbohydrates	Simple Sugar	Glucose Fructose	Lactos Galactose	Sucrose Maltose
			Complex Carbohydrates	Starch	Glycogen	Cellulose
		Fats	Saturated	Cholesterol		
			Unsaturated	Monounsaturated		
				Polyunsaturated	Omega 3 Omega 6	
		Protein	Non Essential Amino Acids			
			Essential Amino Acids	Histidine Isoleucine Leucine	Lycine Methionine Phenylalanine	Threonine Tryptophan Valine
	NON-CALORIES	Water				
		Vitamins	Vitamin A Vitamin C Vitamin D Vitamin E Vitamin K	Bioflavonoids (Vitamin P) B complex Vitamins Thiamine (B$_1$) Riboflavin (B$_2$) Niacon (B$_3$) Pantothenic Acid (B$_5$)	Pyridoxine (B$_6$) Biotin (B$_7$) Folic Acid (B$_9$) Cyanocobalamin (B$_{12}$) Pangamic Acid (B$_{15}$) Choline Inositol PABA	
		Minerals	Calcium Chlorine Chromium Coblat Copper Fluorine Iodine	Iron Magnesium Manganeses Molybdenum Nickel Phosphorus Potassium	Selenium Sodium Sulfur Vanadium Zinc	

The most common definition of FTT is a child whose weight is less than the third to fifth percentile for age on more than one occasion, or whose weight measurements fall two major percentile lines using the standard growth charts of the National Center for Health Statistics (NCHS). The incidence of FTT is highest in children with prematurity and with other medical conditions (Cole & Lanham, 2011).

A diagnosis of "failure to thrive" is designated by a physician. Often, the infant or toddler is referred for a feeding evaluation, a gastrointestinal consult, and/or a nutritional consult.

It is important to rule out a metabolic, gastrointestinal, or autoimmune disorder in a child who is not gaining weight, or has fallen off the growth curve. Most often, the feeding therapist is called in after organic causes are ruled out; however, it is the speech/language pathologist's and/or occupational therapists' ethical responsibility to ensure that a differential diagnosis is established prior to initiating a program plan. The chapter on assessment (6) addresses these issues in the case history portion under diagnostic procedures.

Failure to thrive can occur from some organic, or biological diseases such as, but not limited to:

- Crohn's disease
- Malabsorption disorders
- Irritable Bowel Syndrome
- Genetic anomalies, such as Down Syndrome
- Severe hypotonia
- Severe food allergies
- Pyloric Stenosis
- Reflux Disease/GERD
- Structural deficits, such as Cleft Palate
- HIV infection
- Neonatal Lupus
- Renal Disease
- Congenital Heart Defect
- Celiac Disease

Nonorganic FTT is a condition resulting from adverse environmental or psychosocial factors. This condition most often occurs in areas with poor economic conditions, teen pregnancies, or in children whose birth mothers suffered from malnutrition and/or eating disorders. It is associated with intrauterine growth retardation and overall poor prenatal care. In rare cases, non-organic FTT could be related to a poor bonding between the mother and child, especially if the mother suffers from depression or a mental disease. Non-organic FTT may result from:

- Poverty
- Dysfunctional family interactions (especially maternal depression or drug use)
- Difficult parent-child interactions

- Lack of parental support (e.g., no friends, no extended family)
- Lack of preparation for parenting
- Family dysfunction (e.g., divorce, spouse abuse, chaotic family style)
- Difficult child (prior to this characterization, the provider should seek out explanations as to why, including subtle dysphagia)
- Child neglect
- Emotional deprivation syndrome
- Poor feeding or feeding skills disorder
- Feeding disorders (e.g., anorexia, bulimia)

Most often, non-organic FTT is of interest to speech-language pathologists and occupational therapists when it is concurrent with oral motor disorders and/or sensory issues. Nonorganic FTT can also result in self-limited diets, which can be addressed in a sensory-motor feeding program.

Tube Feedings

Tube feedings are prescribed in cases of severe FTT. There are several types of tube feedings. The first, a nasogastric feeding tube, or "NG-tube", is passed through the nares (nostril), down the esophagus and into the stomach. This type of feeding tube is generally recommended to address short-term feeding issues, preferably not to exceed 2-4 months. Unfortunately, NG tubes are often used for longer periods of time, which contributes to sensory-motor feeding disorders. NG tubes disrupt the normal suck swallow-breathe process (Bartlett & Werner, 2006).

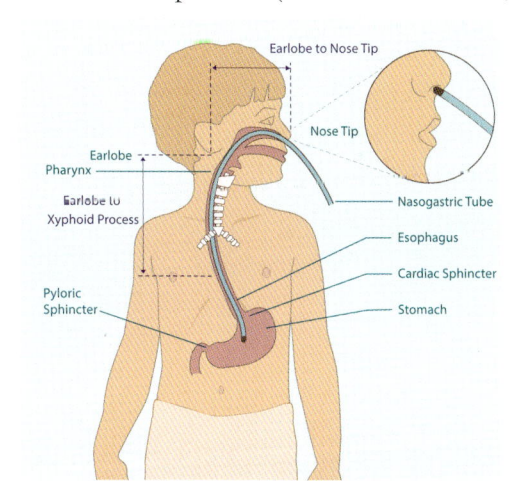

A gastric feeding tube, G-tube or "button," is a tube inserted through a small incision in the abdomen into the stomach and is used for long-term enteral nutrition. One type is the percutaneous endoscopic gastrostomy (PEG) tube. It is placed endoscopically. The patient is sedated and an endoscope is passed through the mouth and esophagus into the stomach. The site of delivery for enteral feedings varies depending on the client's gasterointesinal issues. Less common placement could include Oral-Gastric (OG), Jejunum (J tube) or a Gastric-Jejunum (G-J) Tube.

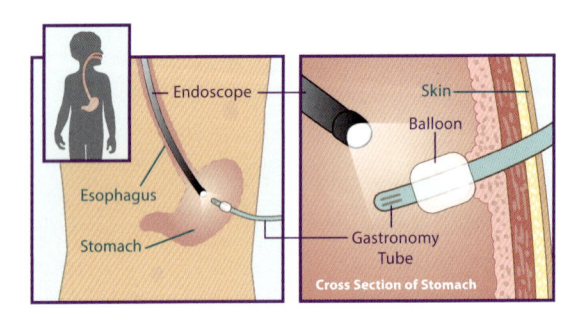

A speech-language pathologist is often consulted for advice regarding tube feedings as part of an overall feeding and nutrition plan. When there are adequate or improving oral sensory-motor skills, the speech/language pathologist will undoubtedly want to move toward oral feeding as soon as it is medically cleared (ASHA, 2009).

Challenges can result when other professionals want to maintain a certain calorie goal through bolus feeding. For example, physicians and dietitians may not agree on when feedings should occur. Quite often, children are fed at night while they are sleeping, and oral-phase feeding therapy is conducted during the day (Fucile, Gisel & Lau, 2002). This can be problematic in terms of hunger and satiation. The night feeding teaches the brain to accept food in the night hours as opposed to day, compromising hunger levels during waking hours. It is suggested that bolus feeds occur during the day to coincide with the sensations of hunger and satiation.

Subclinical Nutritional Deficiencies

A critical problem in working with children with feeding disorders is that long term deprivation of nutrients can impact growth, bone health, and organ efficiency (Dorfman, n.d.). Self-limited diets often lack protein, fiber, and natural nutrients. Oral sensory-motor disorders can make many foods difficult to masticate and swallow, and limit the intake of the quantity of foods needed to thrive. Over the long term, the combination of these issues can cause a variety of nutritional deficiencies that include:

1. Calcium deficiency
   - Osteoporosis
   - Rickets
   - Tetany
2. Iodine deficiency
   - Goiter
3. Selenium deficiency
   - Keshan disease
4. Iron deficiency
   - Iron deficiency anemia
5. Zinc
   - Growth retardation
6. Thiamine (Vitamin B1)
   - Beriberi
7. Niacin (Vitamin B3)
   - Pellagra
8. Vitamin C
   - Scurvy
9. Vitamin D
   - Osteoporosis
   - Rickets

While nutritive oral feedings may be the goal, there are often difficult decisions along the way when deciding between enteral feeds, oral feeds, or a combination of both (Arvedson & Brodsky, 2001).

Vitamin & Mineral Supplements

Vitamins and minerals are important elements of the total nutritional requirements for children. Because the human body itself is unable to produce adequate amounts of many vitamins, they must be obtained from the diet. The body needs these vitamins in only tiny amounts, and in a balanced diet they are usually present in sufficient quantities in the foods a person eats. Thus, individuals with feeding disorders may not get sufficient quantities of vitamins and minerals from their diets (Arvedson & Brodsky, 2001).

For some children, pediatricians may recommend a daily supplement. This may occur as a result of poor appetite, erratic eating habits, or self-limited diets. A vitamin supplement is usually considered. Chewable tablets are available for children who have difficulty swallowing pills. Compounding pharmacies offer liquid alternatives for those children who cannot chew tablets. A common problem, however, is that many children with special needs will not accept vitamins even in a chewable or liquid form.

Supplementation of vitamins and minerals has been found to be very beneficial for children with limited diets and feeding disorders. The first step is a simple blood test to assess vitamins in the system such as B, D, and A. The physician can then determine what, if any, vitamins and minerals may be deficient. Children with specific nutritional deficits (e.g., lack of vitamin D), may be given specific supplements as opposed to a general multivitamin.

Specific vitamins seem to support various systems of human organs and brain function. There seems to be a correlation between nutritional deficiencies and low muscle tone (Dorfman, n.d.). Minerals and supplements can be used to support behavior management, calmness, digestion and the development of the brain (Boyle & Yeargin-Allsopp, 1994). For example, women are now urged to take prenatal vitamins with folic acid and DHEA in the pre-conception phase. Folic acid is taken to reduce the changes of spina bifida in the fetus. Essential fatty acids are often recommended and taken to aid in the fetus's brain development.

The following are examples of specific vitamins and minerals and how they relate to body function and immune support:

VITAMIN ANTIVIRAL	ANTIBACTERIAL PROPERTIES
Vitamin A (beta-carotene)	Supports the immune system
Vitamin B complex	Supports the immune system, helps with digestion of fats and carbohydrates, improves concentration, memory, balance, and helps maintain stability of the central nervous system
Vitamin B6 + magnesium	Improves attention, responsiveness, play, appetite, speech development, cooperation, bladder control. Reduces moodiness, frustrations, temper tantrums, and hyperactivity
Vitamin C	Supports immune system, reduces allergy symptoms, and has anti-viral, anti-bacterial properties
Choline	Increases memory for learning, assists liver function
Magnesium Oxide	Helps promote typical heart rhythm

Fish Oils/DHEA	Helps support brain and speech development
Calcium + Magnesium + Vitamin D	Promotes healthy teeth and bones
Vitamin E	Active antioxidant
Folic Acids	Helps metabolize protein and maintains cell division
Selenium	An active antioxidant that supports the immune system
Zinc	Important for brain function, improves mental alertness
Amino Acids (L-Carnatine, L-Glutamine, L-Taurine, L-Gluathione)	Important in the metabolism of fat, removes toxins, detoxifying, reduces indigestion and ulcers
Essential fatty Acids (Omega ^, Omega 3)	Chemical building blocks for fat that cannot be produced by the body. They are critical for the immune system
Probiotics	Aids in digestion and helps support the immune system

(This chart was compiled using information from www.answers.com, www.netwellness.com and www.wikipedia.com)

There are some nutritionists and integrative physicians, such as Kelly Dorfman, M.S. LDN, Kenneth Bock M.D, and James A. Neubrander, M.D., who believe diets and supplements can decrease behaviors and stereotypes associated with autism. Vitamin and mineral regimens are often paired with therapeutic diet plans. This leads us to our next topic on specialized diets. More information can be found through the Autism Research Institute (www.autism.com).

Specialized Diets

Over the past five years, there has been increased awareness of how diets can impact the behaviors and general well-being of children who present with Autism Spectrum Disorder (ASD) and Pervasive Developmental Disorder. Digestive issues are common among children with autism.

Symptoms ranging from abdominal distention to abnormal stool appearance are often reported (Kuddo & Nelson, 2003).

Some physicians believe that many children with ASD suffer from "leaky gut syndrome," a disease in which a damaged intestine is caused by the insufficient breakdown of food particles, and that this causes leakage of these particles into the bloodstream (Gottschall, 1994). Leaky Gut is also associated with the overgrowth of yeast. The yeast that develops slowly causes secondary symptoms including: diarrhea, constipation, and ulcerations of the intestinal walls. Leaky gut has also been associated with autoimmune diseases, Celiac Disease, Chronic Fatigue, Crohn's Disease, anxiety, asthma, arthritis, and liver problems. Secondary symptoms include decreased attention, atypical sensory reactions, skin rashes, mood swings, and migraine headaches (Balzola et al., 2005; Gonzalez et al., n.d.; Horvath et al., 1999; Kuddo & Nelson, 2003).

With increased awareness of the gastrointestinal issues associated with ASD, pioneers in integrative medicine joined through a group entitled "Defeat Autism Now" (DAN). DAN completes research and clinical trials to evaluate the connection between autism and GI issues. The DAN movement has been the major force behind the emergence of Gluten and Casein Free (GFCF) diets for children on the autism spectrum (Balzola et al., 2006). Gluten is the mixture of proteins, including gliadins and glutelins (found in wheat grains), which are not soluble in water and which give wheat dough its elastic texture. Casein is a white, tasteless, odorless protein precipitated from milk by rennin.

Example of a GFCF diet is as follows:

SAFE	UNSAFE
Fruits	Milk products
Vegetables	Butter
Dried fruits	Wheat
Coconut	Bulgar
Rice products	Barley
Nuts	Soy sauce
Fresh meats	Starches
Fresh fish	Malt
Quinoa products	Regular pasta
Potato products	Couscous
Corn Products	Oats
Eggs	Rye
Beans	Semolina
Lentils	Whey
Buckwheat, Millet and Soy	Lactose

Some parents, doctors and researchers have stated that children have shown mild to dramatic improvements in speech and/or behavior after these substances were removed from their diets. Some also report that their children have experienced fewer bouts of constipation and diarrhea since starting a gluten-free, casein-free (GFCF) diet (Balzola et al., 2006; Merkel-Walsh, 2012). Following a GFCF has its pros and cons. Availability of products is dependent on geographic location.

The Specific Carbohydrate Diet (SCD™) is another nutritional resource for children with ASD. The SCD™ is based on the premise that limiting the diet to simple sugars (usually for at least a year) will starve out toxic organisms in the gastrointestinal (GI) tract and restore gut integrity and immune function. It is a diet intended mainly for Crohn's disease, ulcerative colitis, Celiac disease, diverticulitis, cystic fibrosis, and chronic diarrhea. Like the GFCF diet, DAN doctors and nutritionists support the use of the SCD™ (Merkel-Walsh, 2012).

Some general guidelines of the SCD™ are: no grains (i.e., rice, wheat, corn, oats, etc.), no processed foods, no starchy vegetables (i.e. potatoes, yams, etc.), and no canned vegetables of any kind, no flour, no sugar, no sweeteners other than honey and Stevia, and no milk products except for homemade yogurt fermented for 24 hours. This diet is far more restrictive than the GFCF diet; however, parent testimonials have been very positive for the reduction of autism behaviors and stereotypies.

Food Allergies/Sensitivities

Food allergies/sensitivities are becoming much more common in children. As many as eight percent of the general population suffers from food allergies. The American Academy of Pediatrics (AAP) debate why food allergies are on the rise. Some suggested theories include: pollution of our environment and food sources or increases in clinical diseases. Others attribute it to greater awareness by physicians and other health care providers, as well as parents (Fasano, 2011). The most common food allergies are milk, eggs, nuts, soy, wheat and shellfish (FAAN, 2012).

> **FOOD ALLERGIES ARE ON THE RISE**

The earliest signs of food allergies/sensitivities may begin at birth when an infant has adverse reaction to formula or breast milk. Symptoms include: vomiting, reflux, eczema, failure to thrive, atypical stools, and skin rashes. More severe reactions, such as anaphylactic shock includes: swelling of the throat, difficulty breathing and swelling of the lips and tongue. These reactions can be life threatening. Less common food allergy symptoms are: geographic tongue, abnormal raised patches on the hard palate, redness of the ears, and mouth sores (Bahr, 2010).

If a member of the feeding team suspects food allergies/sensitivities in a child, an allergist can perform a variety of tests, to determine food allergies/sensitivities. Skin prick tests and blood tests may determine food allergies. Stool samples and endoscopic studies are also used, especially in infants when skin and allergy tests can be unreliable. IgG blood testing will usually show food intolerances or sensitivities as opposed to anaphylactic reactions.

For infants, some hypoallergenic formulas are available. Since breast feeding is dependent on maternal diet control, the mother may need to avoid all foods that the infant is allergic to. An elimination diet can be used with breast feeding mothers. Rotation of formulas can be used for very sensitive infants (Bahr, 2010). As the infant ages, the parents have to regulate the foods in a child's diet. Quite often the members of the feeding team are actively involved in transitioning infants to a hypoallergenic formula, and/or working with a collaborative team to ensure nutritive feedings and positive growth.

One of the more common food allergies is gluten, and this is called Celiac Disease (CD) Celiac disease is a lifelong inherited autoimmune condition affecting children and adults. When people with CD eat foods that contain gluten, it creates an immune-mediated toxic reaction that causes damage to the small intestine and does not allow food to be properly absorbed. Even small amounts of gluten in foods can affect those with CD and cause health problems. Damage can occur to the small bowel even when there are no symptoms present. Children with CD cannot have gluten, and this needs to be considered when designing a feeding plan. The Celiac Disease Foundation offers support to clients and their families in finding gluten-free foods.

On a final note, individuals with severe seasonal allergies, known as "hay fever," may also have adverse reactions to certain foods, especially during allergy season. This is called "Oral Allergy Syndrome". Considerations must be given to food choices when working with a child who has known ragweed, pollen, and/or grass allergies (Osterweil, 2012).

ORAL ALLERGY SYNDROME

Ragweed Allergy: Ragweed cross-reacts with bananas and melons, so people with ragweed allergies may also react to honeydew, cantaloupe, and watermelons, or tomatoes. Zucchini, sunflower seeds, dandelions, chamomile tea, and Echinacea may also affect some people.
Birch Pollen Allergy: People with birch pollen allergies may react to kiwi, apples, pears, peaches, plums, coriander, fennel, parsley, celery, cherries, carrots, hazelnuts, and almonds.
Grass Pollen Allergy: People with grass allergy may react to peaches, celery, tomatoes, melons, and oranges.

Supplementary Calorie Intake

When working with children who have one or more of the aforementioned issues, the feeding team is often involved in helping with the concentration of calories in foods. Clients with compromised oral sensory-motor skills often cannot handle large amounts of food and liquid so it is very important to ensure that feedings are maximizing calories. Some effective strategies that may be recommended by a nutritionist or dietitian are as follows:

Liquids: Concentrate intake by using more formula powder when preparing a feeding. For example, if the normal dose is 1 scoop of formula powder to 2 ounces of water, use 1.5 scoops of formula powder to 2 ounces of water. Protein powders are also helpful and can now be found with or without gluten and/or casein.

Purees: Add Medium Chain Triglycerides (MCT) oil (fats found in palm and coconut oils), polycose, vegetable oil, wheat germ, powdered milk, avocado, protein powder, butter, whole milk, coconut milk, pureed beans, supplemental toddler formulas (e.g., Neocate Nutra, Duocal), and cheese.

Examples: Cream of Wheat cereal with butter, wheat germ + whole milk, apple sauce with cinnamon + Duocal.

Solids: Add coconut oil, olive oil, nut butters, creamy dips, hummus, melted cheese, butter.

Examples: Instead of plain crackers, add almond butter. In a turkey sandwich, add hummus.

Additional strategies for diet shaping will be discussed in Chapter 10.

Food and Drug Interactions

The Food and Drug Administration (FDA) often warns patients of food and drug interactions on pharmaceutical labels; however, the treating therapist may not always have access to these labels. It is important to research possible food and drug interactions with each specific case. When taking a case history (see Chapter 6), the therapist/family must be sure to list all medications a client is taking, along with any nutritional supplements. Several factors must be considered when designing a program plan for feeding:

- Medications may need to be taken at different times relative to meals
- Medications can interact with nutrients in food
- Nutritional supplements can interact with medications
- Medications should always be taken with water unless otherwise advised
- The doctor should determine the best time of day to take the medications
- The form of the medication (e.g., some medications can be crushed while others cannot)

The following are examples of food/drug interactions (FDA, n.d.):

Grapefruit juice: Grapefruit juice is often mentioned as a product that can interact negatively with drugs, but the actual number of drugs the juice can interact with is less well-known. That's because grapefruit juice can cause higher levels of those medicines in your body, making it more likely that you will have side effects from the medicine.

Licorice: This would appear to be a fairly harmless snack food. Licorice can reduce the effects of blood pressure drugs or diuretic (urine-producing) drugs, including Hydrodiuril (hydrochlorothiazide) and Aldactone (spironolactone).

Chocolate: Monoamine Oxidase (MAO) inhibitors are just one category of drugs that shouldn't be consumed with excessive amounts of chocolate. The caffeine in chocolate can also interact with stimulant drugs such as Ritalin (methylphenidate), increasing their effect, or by decreasing the effect of sedative-hypnotics such as Ambien (zolpidem.)

Foods with Vitamin K: Spinach, cauliflower, brussel sprouts, potatoes, vegetable oil, and egg yolk all can be very dangerous when mixed with anticoagulant medications such as Coumadin.

Milk and dairy products: Certain antibiotics such as Tetracycline, Hydrochloride and Achromycin should not be taken within two hours of consuming dairy products or taking a calcium supplement.

Similar interactions between nutritional supplements and drugs

Vitamin E: Taking vitamin E with a blood-thinning medication such as Coumadin can increase anti-clotting activity and may cause an increased risk of bleeding.

Ginseng: This herb can interfere with the bleeding effects of Coumadin. In addition, ginseng can enhance the bleeding effects of heparin, aspirin, and nonsteroidal anti-inflammatory drugs such as Ibuprofen, Naproxen, and Ketoprofen.

Ginkgo Biloba: High doses of the herb Ginkgo Biloba could decrease the effectiveness of anticonvulsant therapy in patients taking the following medications to control seizures: Tegretol, Equetro, or Carbatrol (carbamazepine), and Depakote (valproic acid).

This list is far from complete, but provides good examples of the types of interactions that could be present when working with a child who has a feeding disorder.

When to consult with a nutritionist

In this chapter, we have defined many important factors related to a client's optimal nutrition. The feeding therapist is responsible for determining types of food used in therapy and their reactions and relationship to general nutrition, and interaction with medications and supplements. Food allergies/sensitivities and specialized diets must also be considered.

While a feeding therapist may have knowledge in these areas, in many cases a nutritionist or dietitian, will be consulted regarding a child's specific nutritional needs. Clinical dietitians provide nutritional services to patients in hospitals, nursing care facilities, and other institutions. They assess patients' nutritional needs, develop and implement nutrition programs, and evaluate and report the results. They also confer with doctors and other healthcare professionals to coordinate medical and nutritional needs.

Nutritionists can collaborate on feeding program plans by helping the feeding team set caloric goals. They can suggest substitutions for foods when there are allergies, calculate average daily caloric intake, analyze drug and food interactions, and balance foods from various food groups (proteins, starches, etc.)

CONCLUSION:

Speech-language pathologists on a feeding team need to understand basic nutrition. Failure to Thrive (FTT), tube feedings, subclinical nutritional deficiencies, vitamins and supplements, specialized diets, and food allergies/sensitivities may be factors which impact an oral sensory-motor feeding disorder. Co-treatment and collaboration with nutritionists and dietitians are critical for client care.

CHAPTER 5:
SENSORY PROCESSING – A SIMPLIFIED SUMMARY

LEADING GOALS/POINTS

Understanding sensory processing

Recognizing sensory processing dysfunction as it relates to feeding

Identifying characteristics of sensory modulation disorders as they relate to feeding

Identifying characteristics of sensory discrimination disorders

Identifying characteristics of sensory based motor disorders

Imagine you are spoon-feeding a typically developing 9-month-old baby. You present a new food. The baby clears the food off the spoon, his eyes open wide, and he moves the food around his mouth, looks curiously at you as if to say, "What did you just give me?" He may lean forward and open his mouth again or lean back and close his mouth while he tries to decide if he wants more of this new food. This is a typical reaction.

A baby with sensory processing issues may have a totally different reaction. In response to the new food, the baby may start screaming, rubbing his tongue, gagging, and possibly even vomit. Any attempt to reintroduce this food may result in his pushing the food away or crying hysterically. This baby's response certainly was "mismatched" with the input.

The goal of this chapter is not to present a comprehensive view of sensory processing disorders. Instead it will present a simplified summary that will allow the reader to understand how sensory processing issues impact the oral sensory-motor phase of feeding.

Self Regulation and Arousal

The newborn baby seeks comfort through sucking, swaddling, or listening to the mother's heartbeat. In the first three months of life, infants learn to regulate their state. This allows them to calm themselves and become attentive to their world.

Arousal is the level of alertness that allows us to prepare for any activity. State regulation allows for adequate arousal. It is arousal that allows an infant to be in touch with his/her new world (Bahr, 2001).

Difficulty with self-regulation and/or arousal is often a red flag for developmental disorders. Babies who cannot self-regulate often have difficulty with breast and bottle feeding. Children who are over- or under-aroused may not be able to organize themselves for feeding (Morris & Klein, 1987).

Sensory Processing

Sensory processing describes our ability to take in information from our internal environment and the world around us, organize this information, and use it to respond in a well-regulated way. Difficulty taking in or making sense of sensory input can manifest into behavioral, learning, feeding, emotional, and self esteem problems (Roche et al., 2011).

Occupational Therapists (OTs) are primarily responsible for diagnosing sensory processing dysfunction. The OT who specializes in sensory processing disorders evaluates a child and looks at the various sensory areas that may be impacted. These include the following systems: vestibular, proprioceptive, tactile, auditory, visual, olfactory, (smell) and gustatory (taste). Within each of these systems, they assess modulation and discrimination.

Children with sensory processing issues may present with one or more of the following issues related to the oral-phase of feeding:

- Decreased ability or inability to tolerate smells in the environment to include food
- Decreased ability or inability to handle the sights or sounds in the kitchen or dining area
- Decreased ability or inability to tolerate the sound of chewing

- Decreased ability or inability to sit at the table for mealtimes (may eat better moving around the house)
- Self-limited diet based on taste, texture, temperature, color, smell, or brand
- Decreased ability to control saliva and decreased awareness of saliva on the lips or chin
- Decreased ability to feel food in the mouth and decreased awareness of remaining food in the mouth or on the lips
- Decreased ability to discriminate hunger and satiation (e.g., child who is never hungry)
- Swallows food that is not adequately broken down
- Has food in the mouth for long periods of time, even after it is adequately masticated and ready to swallow
- Will put any non-food item in his/her mouth but will not put food in his/her mouth
- Has a complicated routine related to mealtime
- Decreased motor skills necessary to break down food effectively, resulting in gagging and choking

Sensory Processing Dysfunction

Sensory processing dysfunction is an umbrella term that includes three primary diagnostic categories: 1) sensory modulation disorders; 2) sensory discrimination disorders and 3) sensory-based motor disorders. These diagnostic categories are not mutually exclusive. Differential diagnosis should be done by an OT who specializes in sensory processing disorders.

   1. Sensory Modulation Disorders:

People with sensory modulation disorders have difficulty regulating the nature and intensity of their responses to sensory input. Within this diagnostic category are the subcategories of: sensory over-responsivity, sensory under-responsivity, and sensory seeking/craving. These disorders can relate to feeding issues in the following ways:

Sensory Over-Responsivity:
Children with feeding disorders, who are over-responsive to input, may have strong aversive reactions to various input such as: sound, smell, taste, or texture.

> **FOOD REFUSAL OFTEN HAS A SENSORY BASIS**

Sound:
There are typical sounds in a kitchen, which are background noise to people with intact sensory systems. We hear the sounds but they do not distract us from cooking, eating, or interacting with our friends or family. However, imagine that sounds such as those made by the microwave, blender, dishwasher, toaster oven, food processor, tea kettle, coffee pot; hum of the lights, sound of a knife chopping, silverware clinking, glasses put on the table; or the sound of people chewing (or your own chewing) were so aversive that they were painful to the ears. Your reaction might be to cover your ears, totally shut down, or refuse to eat. You might become so agitated that you have a behavioral response such as humming, crying, or throwing a tantrum.

Smell:
Think about walking into the house and smelling cookies baking, a turkey in the oven, or soup cooking on the stovetop. For most of us, this is a pleasurable experience. If the smell is something we like, it may make us salivate and trigger our appetite. On the other hand, think about smells that are aversive to you personally. These may include: an overly-perfumed seatmate on a long flight, a dirty diaper, or garbage rotting on a hot city street. Just imagining smells can make you gag. For many of the children we work with, this "gag" reaction happens when mom is eating a salad, dad is having cheese and crackers, or when they walk into a kitchen when dinner is cooking.

Taste:
Most of us enjoy a variety of food tastes. When there is something we do not like, we can appropriately refuse that food. Children with sensory processing issues may have a very limited repertoire of foods they can tolerate. Food refusal may be accompanied by gagging, vomiting, and/or adamant avoidance.

Tactile:
Children who have difficulty regulating their responses to tactile input may have aversive reactions to toothbrushing or having their faces touched, wiped, or washed. Additionally they may avoid touching food with their hands or having it in their mouths. It is important to acknowledge the interaction of the sensory and motor systems when it comes to handling food texture. For example, a child's acceptable foods may include purees such as yogurt and crunchy foods such as high taste chips and cookies. The same child may refuse fruits, vegetables, and meats. This child is seeking increased taste and proprioceptive input, but may not have the motor skills to break down chewy textures. If you have had the experience of gagging or choking on a texture you have not managed properly, you may have refused the food the next time it was offered (Toomey & Sundseth Ross, 2011).

Vision:
Over-responsivity to visual input may result in a child self-limiting his/her diet to white, beige, or brown foods or limiting the brand of chicken nuggets, cookies, chips, or yogurt, based on packaging.

Vestibular:
Most people enjoy sitting down and enjoying a meal in the company of friends or family. However, some children need to move to be at the optimal level of arousal to tolerate eating. They graze rather than sit and eat a meal. While this behavior (grazing) is explainable, it is not good for weight gain.

Sensory Under-Responsivity:

Sensory-based feeding disorders may have a greater nutritional impact on people who are over-responsive, because people who are under-responsive may eat indiscriminatively. They may seek out strong tastes such as sour, salty, bitter, spicy, or very sweet. They may not have the sensation of hunger or satiation. They may need to smell everything. They may have difficulty with postural stability to support sitting in a chair to eat. They may not feel where the food is in their mouths, and if they can't feel it, they may not be able to handle it safely. Gagging and choking may be secondary to not getting the input about where the food is, what they need to do to adequately manage the food, or when to swallow it.

> **IF YOU DON'T FEEL IT, CAN YOU HANDLE IT SAFELY?**

Sensory Seeking/Craving:

The child who is sensory seeking may inappropriately mouth everything in his/her environment. This includes but is not limited to: toys, clothes, furniture, door knobs, and rocks. They may try to eat non-food items such as paper, play dough, and dirt. They may eat excessive amounts of food and have difficulty feeling full. They may stuff their mouths and choose high taste foods. When a child who is sensory seeking is a picky eater, this is often the result of the interaction between the sensory and motor systems. For example, a child may seek high taste foods, but will only eat crunchy high taste textures secondary to a reduced ability to masticate other textures. What seemingly presents as a self-limited diet is actually an indication of an oral-phase feeding disorder.

2. Sensory Discrimination Disorders:

People with Sensory Discrimination Disorders have difficulty interpreting or distinguishing sensations. Individuals with Sensory Discrimination Disorder may not be able to discriminate tastes (salty vs. sweet) or textures (crunchy vs. chewy). They may not be able to sense hot food from cold foods. They may drool copiously and not feel the drool running down their lips and chins. They may not get the feedback that they need to swallow saliva or, in many cases, food. They may stop chewing with food in their mouths or swallow and be seemingly unaware of residual food on the surface of the tongue. They may be very messy eaters, since they do not feel the food on their lips, cheeks, or chin. They may swallow a bolus that is too large or chew for long periods of time and not know the food is ready to be swallowed. In many cases they cannot identify a food or where it is located in the oral cavity. This can result in food selectivity due to fear of the unknown.

3. Sensory-Based Motor Disorder:

Oral motor development was described in Chapter 2. In short, babies are born with hard-wired synergies called reflexes that support feeding. The synergies develop into integrated sensory-motor skills based upon a child's experiences within the environment. Delays or deviations in muscle tone, posture, and alignment will be reflected in sensory-motor skills that support feeding. Motor planning issues can also significantly impact feeding. In these cases, children may not be able to execute the motor plan needed to masticate, collect a bolus, and swallow. Each time this person eats, it may be as if they are learning to eat over and over again.

SYNERGIES DEVELOP INTO INTEGRATED MOTOR SKILLS

CONCLUSION:

If you are working with clients who have sensory processing issues, it is important for their oral sensory-motor programs to be carried out in conjunction with a sensory diet designed by an occupational therapist (OT). The goal of a sensory diet is to provide input to the system, which helps to maintain an optimal level of arousal throughout the day. This will be especially important when we discuss sensory-based diet shaping in Chapter 8.

CHAPTER 6:
ASSESSMENT

LEADING GOALS/POINTS

Gathering information for an assessment

Conducting an initial interview and reviewing a client's case history

Preparing a supply inventory for the evaluation

An oral sensory-motor feeding assessment helps a therapist design and implement an individualized treatment program. The assessment determines whether a client has the underlying oral sensory-motor skills to support safe, nutritive feeding. This chapter will describe the essential components of conducting a feeding assessment:

1. Case History/Gathering information
2. Assessment of the oral structure
3. Assessment of underlying oral sensory-motor skill development through the use of pre-feeding activities (Chapter 7)
4. Assessment of oral sensory-motor skill during the observation of a nutritive feeding
5. Observation of trial therapeutic feeding techniques (Chapter 9) in order to develop a therapeutic feeding treatment plan (Chapter 10)

1. Gathering Information/Case History:

Prior to meeting with the child, you will need to gather pertinent information to help plan for your assessment. In addition, parents should be instructed on what they will need to bring to the assessment. This includes:

- Pictures of the child from birth, at approximately 6-month intervals (this helps the clinician see if there are changes to the oral musculature over time)

- A video of the child feeding (if the parent suspects there may be difficulty feeding in the session)
- Adaptive seating if utilized at home
- The utensils the child uses for mealtime
- A variety of food textures and tastes including: purees for spoon feeding, crunchy solids, chewy solids, and liquids

Examples of foods include:

Breast or Bottle	Breast Milk, Formula, Milk
Puree and/or spoon feeding	Applesauce, Pudding, Mashed Potatoes, Baby Food, Sorbet, Jell-O®, Yogurt
Crunchy solids	Chips, Thin Pretzels, Apple Slices, Jicama Sticks, Thin Raw Carrots, Veggie Sticks, Cheese Doodles®, Bambas®
Chewy solids	Fruit Leather, Twizzlers®, Bagels, Sandwiches, Chicken or Meat
Strips	Waffles, French Toast, Chicken Tenders, French Fries, Grilled Cheese Sandwiches
Thickener	Simply Thick®, Rice Cereal
Liquid	High Taste Juices such as Lemonade or Cranberry Juice, Apple Juice, Seltzer Water, Bottled Water

Case History

The second step is obtaining background information through a case history. Gather as much information as possible from the parents or caregiver. This should be done in an interview and in written form. This information can be compared to previous evaluations and medical reports, which the parents should be asked to provide. It is important that parents understand that a complete developmental and medical history is essential to understanding a child's feeding issues.

> **COMPARE INFORMATION FROM PREVIOUS EVALUATIONS, AN INTERVIEW, AND THE CASE HISTORY**

FOR CASE HISTORY FORMS, SEE APPENDIX D

Interview

As a part of the case history you are looking for any additional information that may be pertinent in regard to the feeding disorder. After you review the case history form you will want to ask the caregiver questions regarding any inconsistencies found on the form. If the evaluation is being conducted for an adult patient, then you may be asking the client directly.

Examples of pertinent questions are as follows:

1. Tell me about your child's current diet?
2. Tell me about a routine day regarding your child's feeding?
3. Summarize for me your child's feeding history since birth? (this allows the clinician to compare written and verbal history and flag any inconsistencies.)
4. Has anything changed since you filled out the case history?
5. What is your greatest concern regarding your child's feeding?
6. What do you hope to accomplish with this feeding assessment?

When evaluating infants or severely medically compromised children, parents may have records (feeding intake charts, reflux scales, bowel movement records, tube feeding schedule, changes in respiratory status, etc.). If these records are available, obtain them and look for patterns or red flags.

2. Structure

In Chapter 3, craniofacial and structural issues were outlined. It is important that during the assessment, the facial features, the cranium, the intraoral cavity, dental alignment, and the lips, tongue, and jaw are all assessed for symmetry and structural integrity. Use the Oral Motor Feeding Evaluation Checklist in Appendix D to note remarkable observations.

3. Pre-feeding Assessment

Now that you have gathered background information, you are ready to meet with the child and the family.

The first step of the pre-feeding assessment is observation. There is a great deal of information that can be analyzed in regard to the whole body and sensory processing (see Chapter 5). The clinician should be observing:

- **Posture and Alignment:** look at postural stability and how your client moves through the environment. What you see in the body is what you get in the mouth. These observations will help determine the most appropriate seating and support for the evaluation.

- **Sensory Processing:** look at how the child responds to sound, toys, lighting, and tactile input to determine what sensory supports they may need.

- **Clinical Rapport:** look at how quickly the child will interact with the clinician and make determinations regarding how much time needs to be spent on play and social interaction before the pre-feeding tasks can be introduced.

Following this observation you will have information on seating options based on observation of postural stability. You should have a variety of seating options in your facility. If the child has an adaptive seating position for feeding, you should ask the parents or caregiver to bring this to the evaluation. Whenever possible, consult a Physical Therapist for positioning and support suggestions. The following are examples of seating options that the authors use most frequently.

My Brest Friend®:

My Brest Friend® was developed in a laboratory of new moms, babies, and breastfeeding experts who set out to create a pillow whose sole purpose was to answer all the needs of breastfeeding moms and babies.

Breast Feeding Sling:

This tool supports positioning and privacy.

Boppy® Pillow:

The Boppy® Pillow can be used to support the infant during feedings.

Car Seat:

The infant's car seat provides postural support for both pre-feeding and feeding tasks.

Versa Form®:

Versa Form® Pillows provide customized, semi-permanent positioning anywhere contoured support is needed. Pillows are filled with small styrene beads that mold to the individual's body shape when air is extracted. When the valve is released, Versa Form® regains its flexibility and is ready to be shaped again. Forms a firm, uniform support for all parts of the body, reducing risk of pressure points. Used to accommodate structural deformities and help control posture. Shapes and reshapes in seconds. Easy to clean and disinfect.

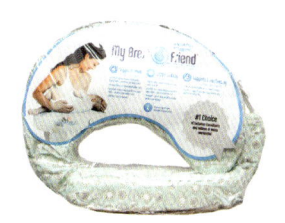

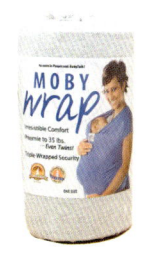

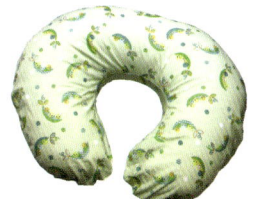

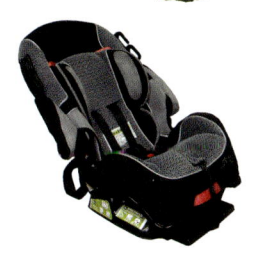

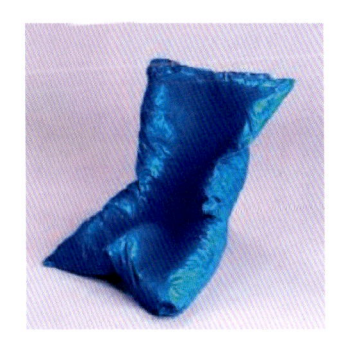

Tumble Form®/Special Tomato®:

Feeder Seats are simple, soft foam positioning seats designed for all ages. They are used for feeding and providing light and portable positioning. They sit on the living room floor or can be held in a parent's lap. They can be put into any stroller and brought to a restaurant setting.

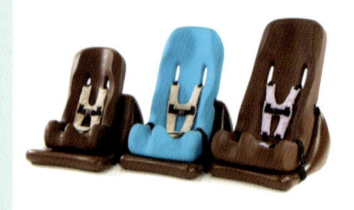

The exclusive coating makes it attractive and easy to wash and maintain. Tumble Form's® seamless covering is washable, odor and stain resistant, impervious to urine, and nontoxic. The contoured interior has a 90-degree seat-to-back relationship to encourage correct seating posture. The small and medium sizes have updated anti-thrust seats for increased pelvic stability. Shoulder harness slots allow 4" of vertical adjustment of the shoulder straps.

First Years® Chair:

This chair is a more affordable and readily available option for parents to use in the home. It provides better head and neck support than most portable booster seats.

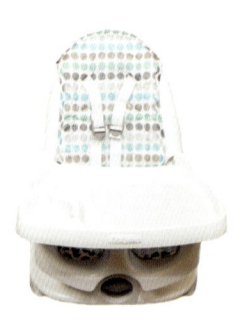

Svan® Highchair:

This chair has adequate supports for pre-feeding and feeding tasks because it is adjustable with a foot rest. The wood design makes it easy to clean, with a variety of washable inserts for comfortable seating. This chair supports the 90-degree angles recommended for therapy.

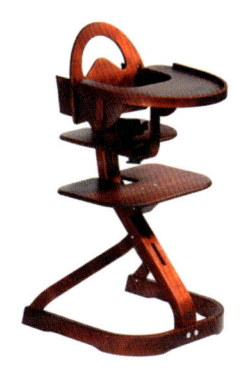

TalkTools® Chair:

Therapists and parents love this chair because it can be adjusted to give supported seating for children ages six months to eight years. It comes with removable cushions to accommodate various sizes and shapes. This chair is constructed of sturdy materials, it has an adjustable footrest for body stability, and a glossy finish for easy cleanup.

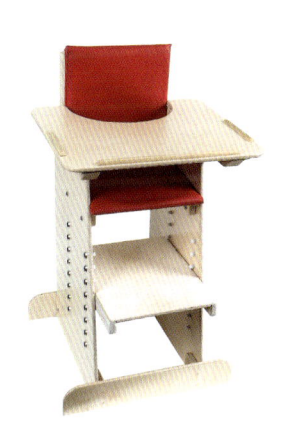

Rifton®:

The Rifton chair is designed to encourage normal, active sitting posture.

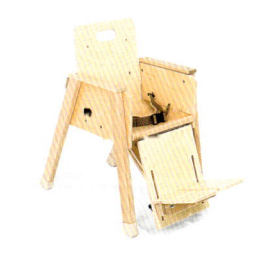

Dycem®:

Placing a piece of Dycem® on the seat of your client's chair will help keep him or her in the correct posture for effective therapy.

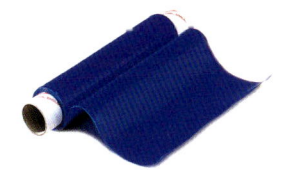

For this part of the assessment a variety of pre-feeding tools will be needed as discussed in detail in Chapter 7. The therapist may need some or all of the following equipment:

Sensory/Pre-Feeding Assessment Tools

(Note: Brief descriptions of tool use are described here. Specific use of the pre-feeding tools will be discussed in Chapter 7.)

Gloves:
Gloves are necessary for protecting both the clinician and the client. Gloves come in a variety of sizes and colors and in latex, non-latex, flavored, and powdered and un-powdered varieties.

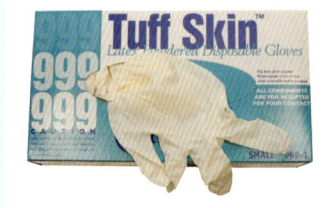

Jiggler (age 1+):
Jigglers add calming and organizing sensory input, and can be used for oral exploration, reducing "fixing" in the jaw, and increasing awareness.

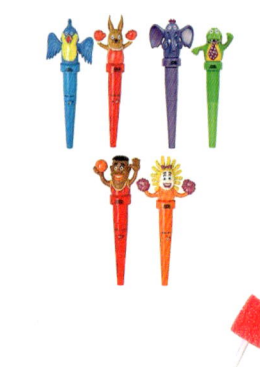

TalkTools® Vibrator and Toothettes® (age 1+):
The hand-held Vibrator & Toothette® provide an excellent option to promote awareness of the oral cavity and to relax "fixing." It is also a valuable tool for diagnosing oral sensitivity.

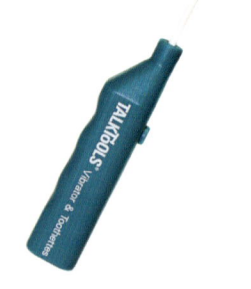

TalkTools® Sensory Bean Bags:
These "bean bags" are a fun and safe way to benefit clients with over-responsive and under-responsive sensory systems. The various textures (silky, bumpy, furry, and scratchy) help normalize sensitivity.

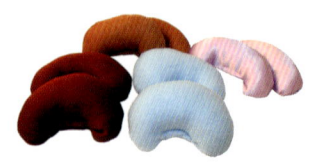

**2 ZVibes® with Spoon Tip,
Green Square Heads, Preefer,
Mouse Head Round Tip,
Fine Tips, and XL Tip:**

This vibrating probe provides an opportunity to increase sensory input during pre-feeding and feeding activities, stimulating increased sensory awareness and mobility in the oral musculature. Various tips are used to achieve different goals. The ZVibe® can also be used in the "off" position for children under one, or for those with seizure disorders.

The **Blue Tip** is the original, designed for older children and adults.

The **Green Mini Tips** are designed for smaller mouths and provide a biting surface for the Chewing Hierarchy found in Chapter 7.

The **Yellow Preefer Tips** are appropriate when a continuous rolling action is desired.

The **Cat-N-Mouse Tip Set** is designed with a variety of textures to generate different sensations within the oral cavity and to the lips and face. Use the ears in your pre-feeding program to facilitate lip closure, or as a spoon for feeding purees. The different textures can be used to encourage oral-sensory exploration.

The **Spoon Tip** can be used to promote lip closure secondary to increased sensory input.

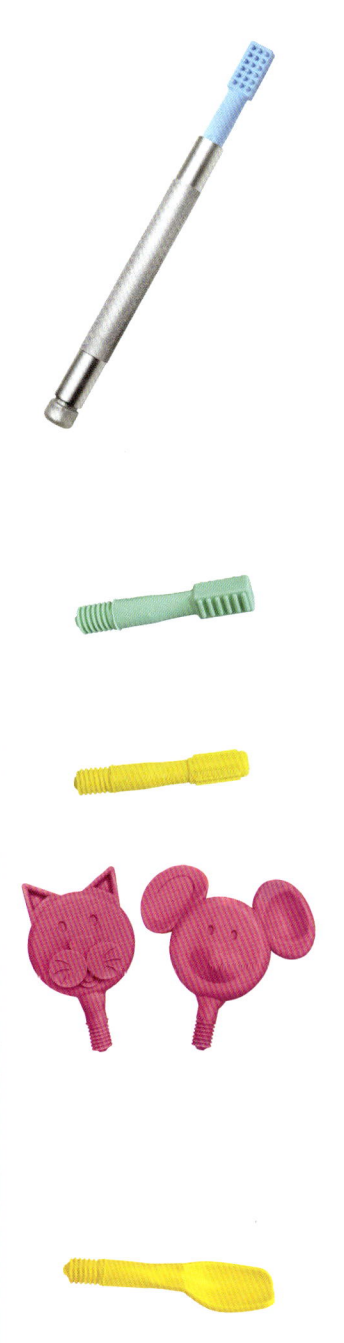

The **Fine Tips** are useful for facilitating tongue elongation and lateralization.

The **XL Bite-n-Chew Head** can be used to add vibration if a Chewy Tube does not provide enough input.

Tips also come in hard or soft, depending on the needs of your client.

Chewy Tubes® (Red and Yellow):
Chewy Tubes are an innovative oral-motor device designed to provide a resilient, non-food, chewable surface for practicing biting and chewing skills, and as an aid to inhibit teeth grinding.

Tongue Depressors:
Tongue Depressors can be used to promote lip closure, nose breathing, and saliva control. They are available in various flavors, as well as non-flavored varieties. Kosher approved tongue depressors are available as well.

Infant Finger Cuff :
The infant finger cuff is smooth on one side with soft rubber bristles on the other. The Finger Cuff can be used to teach the motor plan for chewing. It can also be used to stimulate lateral tongue reflex and oral sensory awareness.

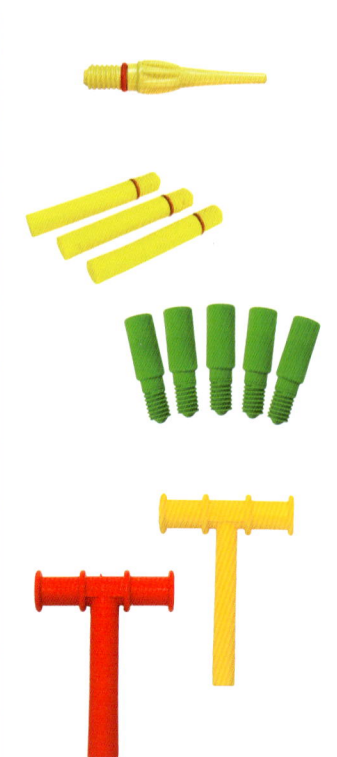

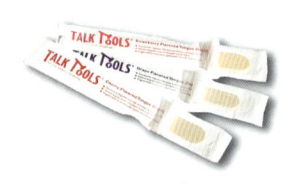

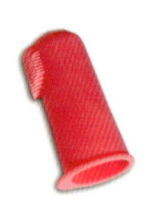

Vibrating Toothbrush:

These tools stimulate lateral molar ridges, the lateral margins of the tongue, and provide sensory input.

Nuk® Massager :

The Nuk® Massager stimulates lateral molar ridges and provides sensory input.

TalkTools® Bite Blocks:

The highly-functional Jaw Grading Bite Blocks promote symmetrical jaw strength and jaw stability. They are helpful in providing jaw stability during pre-feeding tasks described in Chapter 7.

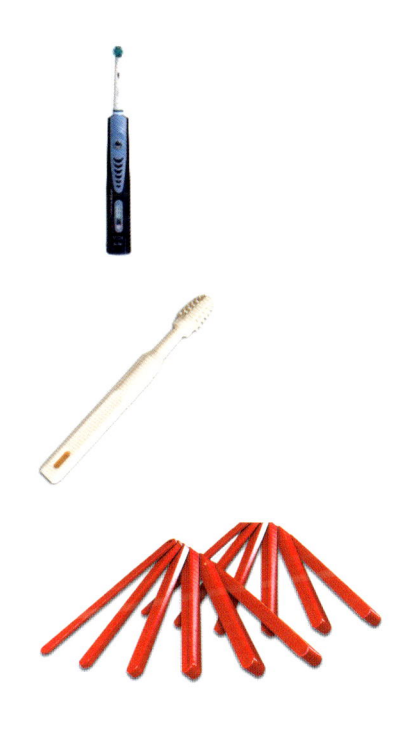

4. Feeding

Ask the caregiver to bring the feeding utensils that the client uses at home. Observe the caregiver feeding the child, or the client eating independently. After observing, implement the therapeutic feeding techniques as described in Chapter 9.

Suggested utensils for feeding may include:

Nipple Shield:
For difficult or persistent latch-on problems, many breastfeeding experts suggest the temporary use of a nipple shield. Made of thin, soft silicone that doesn't interfere with nipple stimulation, the Medela® nipple shield is worn during breastfeeding.

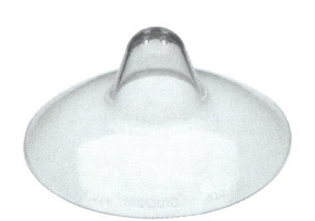

Medela® Haberman Feeder:
This tool has become an essential medical device that is widely used for a variety of feeding difficulties, including cleft lip/palate, neurological dysfunction, congenital heart disease, genetic disorders, and Down Syndrome. It allows infants to bottle and breast feed who have motor planning issues as well as low tone.

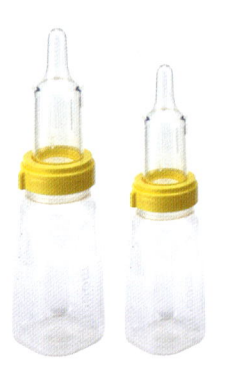

Bag or Vent Bottles:
These bottles are useful for decreasing gas, reflux, and vomiting.

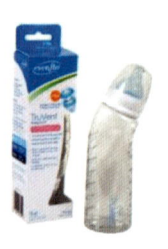

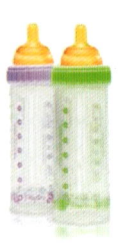

Variety of Nipples:

All infants have different shaped mouths. The size and shape of the nipple impacts labial posture, and the suck-swallow-breathe synchrony. The clinician must have a variety on hand to thoroughly assess bottle feeding.

NON-LATEX/SOFT

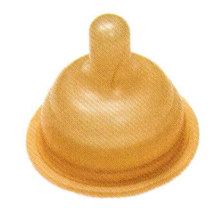

SILCONE/FIRM

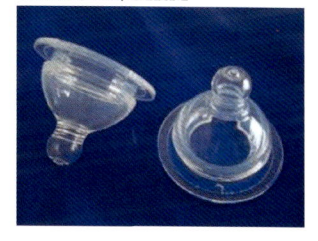

WIDE BASED

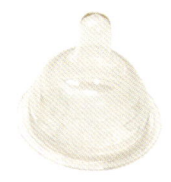

NARROW BASED

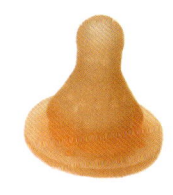

LONG TEAT

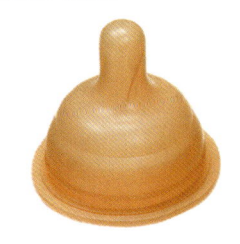

SHORT TEAT

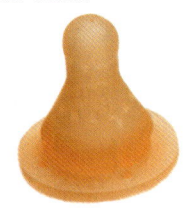

Chapter 6: Assessment

82

Medela® Supplemental Nursing System:
The Supplemental Nursing System enables women to breastfeed who would not otherwise be able to do so. The Supplemental Nursing System is hung around the neck and thin tubes are placed on top of the nipple. The baby cannot feel the tubes during feeding.

Syringe:
Syringes are useful as a supplemental feeding tool.

TalkTools® Honey Bear Cup:
The Honey Bear allows you to control the flow of liquid into a child's mouth and encourages children to learn how to straw drink. It can also be used to transition from bottle-feeding to cup drinking.

TalkTools® Recessed Lid Cup:
The Recessed Lid Cup has two handles to help keep hands at midline, and the recessed lid encourages tongue retraction and improved lip closure. Two twist-off lids are included; can be used for cup or straw drinking.

Cut-Out Cups:
Cut-Out Cups are available in pink (1 oz), blue (2 oz), and green (7 oz). These flexible cups stimulate the corners of the mouth to facilitate lip closure and allow a child to drink without head or neck extension.

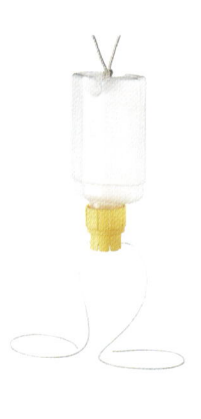

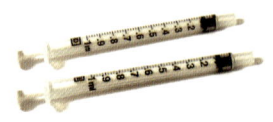

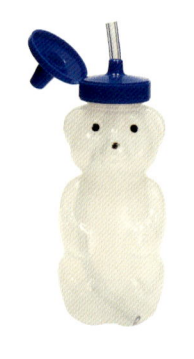

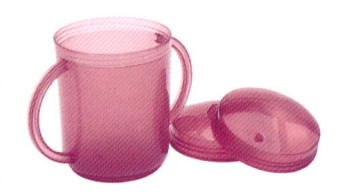

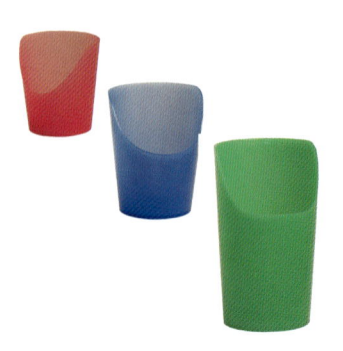

Infa Trainer Cup:

The Infa Trainer Cup allows you to adjust the flow of liquid by twisting the lid, while the design of the lid also allows for stability without encouraging a suckle. This is the preferred alternative to a "sippy cup."

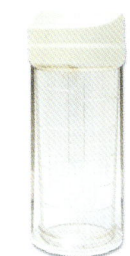

Maroon Spoons:

Maroon Spoons are available in two sizes and promote optimal oral movement and lip closure.

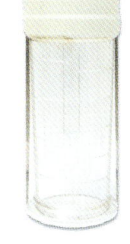

Small Forks and/or Cocktail Forks:

Forks should be appropriate for the size and shape of the client's mouth.

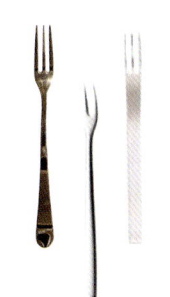

TalkTools® Original Straw Kit:

An excellent supplement to traditional therapy techniques, and the best activity available to promote tongue retraction and controlled tongue movements. The hierarchy promotes jaw-lip-tongue dissociation through twelve stages of development.

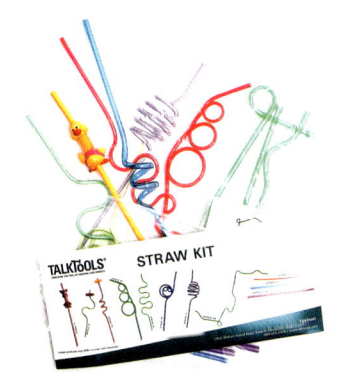

CONCLUSION:

This chapter has outlined what a clinician needs to conduct a pre-feeding and feeding assessment. Gathering information about the client before the assessment is just as important as the observation of the client. Specialized seating, pre-feeding, and feeding tools will be needed at the time of the evaluation. Specific pre-feeding techniques and therapeutic feeding techniques will be discussed in Chapters 7 and 9, respectively.

CHAPTER 7:
A PRE-FEEDING PROGRAM

LEADING GOALS/POINTS

Learning techniques to prepare the oral musculature for feeding

Ensuring safe effective, nutritive feeding

Learning the therapeutic "dance"

Learning to task analyze oral sensory motor skills for feeding

The goal of a pre-feeding program is to develop the motor skills for safe, effective, nutritive feeding. The use of sensory information should be mapped onto your motor goals. Extraneous sensory input, peri- or intra-orally, can be disorganizing as opposed to organizing. As a therapist you must task analyze the motor skills for feeding and ensure that the input you provide is specific to those goals. Prior to introducing oral sensory-motor input, it is essential to ensure that a child is in a balanced state of arousal (Bahr, 2001; Boshart, 2001; Morris & Klein, 2000; Overland, 2011; Rosenfeld-Johnson, 2006). If you cannot touch a child's face, you may need to begin where they can handle the tactile-proprioceptive input. Consultation with an Occupational Therapist as described in Chapter 5 may be warranted.

MAP SENSORY ONTO MOTOR SKILLS

It is important to note that the oral sensory-motor skills for feeding are not always task analyzed by age. Children with deficits in the sensory-motor system may not follow typical norms. Comprehensive description of skills by age can be found in Diane Bahr's text *Oral Motor Assessment and Treatment: Ages and Stages* (2001) and Susan Evans Morris's and Marsha Dunn Klein's text: *Pre-feeding Skills—Second Edition* (2000), which organize pre-feeding tasks by the goals of the motor plan as opposed to the age of the client.

MAINTAINING OPTIMAL AROUSAL

Techniques to Prepare the Oral Musculature

Prior to pre-feeding activities, a child may benefit from tactile, proprioceptive, and/or vestibular input as directed by an Occupational Therapist. Children with sensory processing disorders will benefit from a sensory diet that follows them through life. A sensory diet is well-planned sensory input provided throughout the day with the goal of maintaining an individual's optimal functioning. Examples of sensory input prior to feeding may include: bouncing on a therapy ball, rolling on a scooter board, linear swinging, jumping on a trampoline, deep pressure in a ball pit, Patricia Wilbarger's Brushing Program, use of postural/sensory supports such as a Spio, specific rhythmic music, or rhythmic counting. It may be necessary to present tactile-proprioceptive input on the extremities prior to introducing it on the face or mouth, especially for children who have sensory discrimination issues, or have seizure disorders. Sensory input should be prescribed by an OT who specializes in sensory processing, and it needs to be applied systematically. Therapy can be described as a dance. There is constant interaction between the sensory and the motor systems. It is impossible to separate one from the other. The motor skills used in feeding are carefully choreographed by the therapist. Sensory input is mapped onto motor goals.

THERAPY IS A DANCE

Therapy is also a dance between the child and the therapist or caregiver. If the child pulls back, the therapist needs to pull back. If the client is tolerating sensory-motor input, this provides an opportunity for increasing the demands of therapeutic intervention.

There are critical therapeutic parameters that serve as guidelines for implementation of a pre-feeding program.

1. A pre-feeding program is provided prior to meals or snacks.

2. Touch is firm and elongated. Firm touch is calming.

3. Rate and rhythm is superimposed on oral sensory-motor input, e.g., rhythmic counting, singing, or background music.

4. Input should be graded and repetitive.

5. Sensory information serves to facilitate specific motor goals. The pre-feeding program is specific to the motor skills for feeding.

6. Pre-feeding goals are one step ahead of feeding goals. For example, while a child is being bottle or breast fed, you are working on the oral sensory-motor skills for spoon-feeding or, when the child is eating purees from a spoon, you are working on mastication skills via the chewing hierarchy.

7. Food should not be introduced until the child demonstrates the prerequisite oral sensory-motor skills as outlined in Chapter 2.

8. Pre-feeding activities are based upon task analysis of your client's oral sensory-motor skills.

9. When you introduce a new activity you may need to start in increments of 1-2 repetitions and slowly work up to the desired frequency.

10. The use of cold temperatures can improve sensory processing in clients who have sensory systems that are under-responsive. Cold temperatures can be paired with your pre-feeding tools (e.g., dipping a toothette in ice water).

11. Vibration directly stimulates the proprioceptive system. Many children that we treat are seeking proprioceptive input, even when they dislike tactile input. The use of vibration may be

helpful for both clients with hypotonia and hypertonia. When you initially provide vibration to a muscle, the muscle fires, and muscle function increases. If vibration is sustained over a long period of time, the muscle relaxes. Therefore when using vibration with low tone clients, the input is short and graded. In comparison, if they are able to tolerate it, vibration could be used over a longer period of time with high tone clients. Use vibration cautiously with clients who have seizures or are under a year of age. Always present vibrating tools on the extremities before placing them on or in the oral cavity.

12. If the client requires jaw support for stability during pre-feeding exercises, provide the support with the non dominant hand.

13. At the start of a pre-feeding session, facial massage can be used with any client regardless of their age or tone. The goals of facial massage are to facilitate midline orientation, increase cheek and upper lip mobility while providing increased sensory awareness, and decrease over-sensitivity to oral input. Place two or more fingers or Sensory Bean Bags on the tempromandibular joint (TMJ). Provide firm, elongated massage from the TMJ to the corners of the lips. Reposition your fingers alongside the nose, under the eye socket, and provide firm elongated massage towards the insertion of the upper lip. Reposition your fingers under the nostrils and provide firm elongated massage into the upper lip. Repeat this sequence 4-5 times.

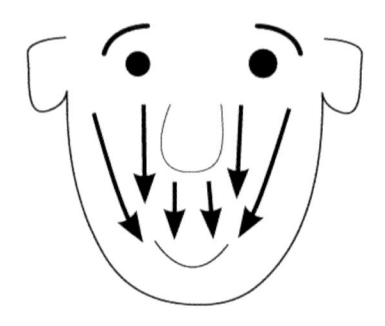

14. If your client has a fixed, retracted, upper lip you can use myofascial release to reduce restriction and allow for neuromuscular reeducation. Sink your fingers into the tissue surface under the nostrils and provide a firm elongated stretch. Your fingers will move through the fascial surface into the muscle insertion of the upper lip. Only one release is needed.

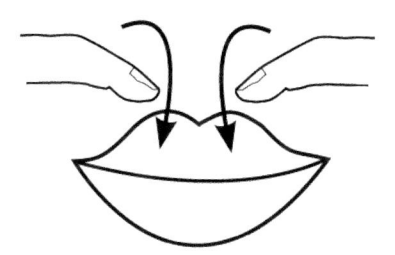

15. If your client has reduced muscle tone, you can use firm rhythmic tapping to increase muscle firing. Provide firm rhythmic tapping from the TMJ to the corners of the lips, and on the surface of the lips to the beat of a favorite song, nursery rhyme or to rhythmic counting.

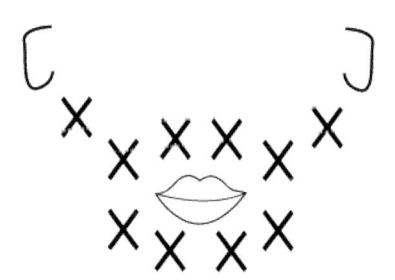

16. Therapeutic intervention that is fun is also reinforcing. A child's work is play. This drives the therapeutic interactions.

17. If you are working with older children or adults, explain the goal of the activity.

Pre-Feeding Activities

SUPPORT ORAL-PHASE SKILL DEVELOPMENT

The pre-feeding activities described are organized to support oral-phase feeding skills for breast and bottle feeding, spoon feeding, mastication of a variety of textures of solid food, as well as straw- and cup-drinking.

Exercises/activities are presented in a hierarchy; therefore, they should be performed in the order listed, going from passive to active. Passive exercises and activities do not require the client to cognitively engage in a motor plan, while active exercises will require volitional movement. Many of the exercises/activities work from peri-orally to intra-orally for clients who are defensive to tactile-kinesthetic input in their mouths.

The number of sets and repetitions are based on the principles of exercise physiology, as well as the necessary units to reinforce a motor plan (O'Sullivan, 2007).

Breast and Bottle Feeding

Pre-requisite skills:

- The coordination of the suck-swallow-breathe synchrony

- Tongue bowling to support the nipple

- An infant orients to the nipple (rooting response), opens the mouth widely (gape response), brings the tongue down to floor of mouth, extends it over the lower lip to grasp the nipple. The mouth closes, the anterior tongue cups to hold the nipple, the body of the tongue grooves to stabilize the nipple. The nipple is enclosed between the grooved tongue, cheeks and palate, forming a teat. The nipple should contact the infant's posterior hard palate. After attachment the infant holds the nipple with the anterior and mid-tongue, with the lips assisting; the soft palate hinges downward, contacting the back of the tongue; the nipple is sealed between the soft palate, grooved tongue, lips, and cheeks. The tongue is grooved from front to back, milk sprays from the nipple and forms a bolus, the soft palate elevates, pharyngeal walls contract (to close off nasal passage), vocal folds are closed by arytenoid cartilage moving together. The epiglottis tilts down to direct milk around vocal folds, suprahyoid muscles pull the larynx upward to shorten the pharynx, and the tongue uses positive pressure to push the bolus of milk into the pharynx for transit to the esophagus (Genna, 2012).

EXERCISE	TARGET GROUPS	GOALS	TOOLS
Palatal massage	0-12 months Hypotonia Hypertonia	Normal development of the palatal vault Sensory awareness	Gloved finger
Place a gloved finger midline on the palatal raphe. Roll your finger out to the lateral ridge (where the infant's teeth will insert) and stop. Replace your finger on the midline raphe, and roll your finger toward the opposite lateral molar ridge. Repeat 5x . If tolerated, 2 sets. The input should be firm, but not hard, and make sure the finger is only on the hard palate.				

EXERCISE	TARGET GROUPS	GOALS	TOOLS
Corner to midline upper lip stretch	Any age Hypotonia Fixed upper lip Hypertonia	Upper lip mobility and strength	Trimmed Toothette (nonflavored) Gloved finger Infadent
Place a gloved finger or a well-trimmed dampened toothette under the upper lip. Roll the tool or finger, from the corner of the lips to midline. Reposition the tool or finger in the opposite corner of the lips and roll to midline. Repeat this sequence 4-5x.				

EXERCISE	TARGET GROUPS	GOALS	TOOLS
Tongue bowling	Infant	Develop the tongue bowl to support the nipple	Gloved finger

Place a gloved finger at the tip of the tongue and provide firm input from the tongue tip towards midline about ¼ of an inch. Reposition finger to the tip of the tongue and repeat 4-5x. Note that 2 sets may need to be completed if the infant does not cup his or her tongue around the finger.

1/4 - 1/2 inch

EXERCISE	TARGET GROUPS	GOALS	TOOLS
Pacifier Rock	Infant	Develop the motor plan for sucking	Rounded pacifier such as the "Soothie" or gloved finger

Place a gloved finger or a pacifier midline on the infant's tongue, so the tongue cups around the tool. Simultaneously place non dominant hand with middle finger under the bony process of the mandible with thumb and pointer finger around the cheeks. As the infant initiates a suck, gently rock the jaw in a forward motion while providing slight resistance to the pacifier or finger. Repeat 4-5x.

Spoon Feeding

Pre-requisite skills:
- Jaw stability and grading
- Upper lip needs to mobilize down and forward
- Lower lip rolls in slightly to stabilize the spoon
- Tongue retraction to facilitate oral transport of the puree
- Contraction through the lateral borders of the tongue
- Contraction in the cheeks to provide the intraoral pressure to support swallowing
- Dissociated tongue tip elevation to initiate a swallow

Pre-feeding activities to achieve these prerequisite skills:

EXERCISE	TARGET GROUPS	GOALS	TOOLS
Jiggler Roll	Any age 1+ Hypertonia Hypotonia	Upper lip mobility	Jiggler
Position the cone-shaped handle of the Jiggler horizontally under the nostrils and roll the Jiggler toward the insertion of the upper lip. Reposition the tool and repeat 4-5x.			

EXERCISE	TARGET GROUPS	GOALS	TOOLS
Mickey Mouse Ears	Any age 1+ Hypertonia Hypotonia	Upper lip mobility Lip closure	ARK's Z-Vibe® with a Mickey Mouse tip head or Ellie the Elephant Jiggler
Place the cupped and textured ear of the Mouse Spoon Tip (or the ear of Ellie elephant) between the child's lips. The vibrating probe will facilitate upper lip mobility into the cupped ear to facilitate the motor plan for spoon feeding.			Stabilize

EXERCISE	TARGET GROUPS	GOALS	TOOLS
Corner to Midline Upper Lip Stretch	Any age Hypotonia Fixed upper lip Hypertonia	Upper lip mobility and strength	Gloved finger, Infadent, Well trimmed toothette, Z-Vibe® yellow preefer head with or without vibration
Place a gloved finger or tool under the upper lip. Roll the tool or finger, from the corner of the lips to midline. Reposition the tool or finger in the opposite corner of the lips and roll to midline. Repeat this sequence 4-5x.			

EXERCISE	TARGET GROUPS	GOALS	TOOLS
Cheek stretch	Any age Passive exercise Hypotonia Hypertonia	Cheek mobility, Lip strength, Lip mobility, Lip rounding, For feeding and speech	Infadent Yellow rounded Z-Vibe® Tip Trimmed Toothette (nonflavored)

Place the tool in the child's cheek and stroke the inside of the cheek from top to bottom in a "C" pattern 4-5x on each side.

EXERCISE	TARGET GROUPS	GOALS	TOOLS
Cheek resistance	Any age Requires active movement Hypotonia Hypertonia	Cheek mobility, Lip strength, Lip mobility, Lip rounding, For feeding and speech	Gloved finger Trimmed toothette Z-Vibe® yellow preefer head with or without vibration

Place a tool inside the cheek approximately where the child would contract the cheeks for sucking (masseter muscle.) Stretch the cheek outward and instruct your client to suck in or give a kiss. Repeat 4-5x on each side.

A Sensory Motor Approach to Feeding

EXERCISE	TARGET GROUPS	GOALS	TOOLS
Lateral tongue massage	Any age 1+	Elongtion of the tongue and tongue lateralization	Trimmed Toothette Z-Vibe® with fine tip *(note: if there is jaw instability use Bite Block level 6 or 7 to stabilize the jaw on the opposite side of the stimulus)*
Stroke the lateral borders of the tongue from back to front 4-5x on one side and then 4-5x on the opposite side for 2 sets.			

Mastication of Solid Foods

Pre-requisite skills:
- Jaw stability
- Jaw grading to bite through a variety of food textures
- Mobility through the tongue tip and lateral borders of the tongue to facilitate oral transport
- Contraction of the cheeks
- Lip closure

Pre-feeding activities to achieve these prerequisite skills:

EXERCISE	TARGET GROUPS	GOALS	TOOLS
Jiggler roll	Any age 1+ Hypertonia Hypotonia	Upper lip mobility	Jiggler
Position the cone-shaped handle of the Jiggler horizontally under the nostrils and roll the Jiggler toward the insertion of the upper lip. Reposition the tool and repeat 4-5x.			

EXERCISE	TARGET GROUPS	GOALS	TOOLS
Corner to Midline Upper Lip Stretch	Any age Hypotonia Fixed upper lip Hypertonia	Upper lip mobility and strength	Gloved finger Infadent Well trimmed toothette Z-Vibe® yellow preefer head with or without vibration

Place a gloved finger or tool under the upper lip. Roll the tool or finger from the corner of the lips to midline. Reposition the tool or finger in the opposite corner of the lips and roll to midline. Repeat this sequence 4-5x.

EXERCISE	TARGET GROUPS	GOALS	TOOLS
Cheek Stretch	Any age Passive exercise Hypotonia Hypertonia	Cheek mobility Lip strength Lip mobility Lip rounding For feeding and speech	Infadent Yellow Z-Vibe® Tip Trimmed Toothette (nonflavored)

Place the tool in the child's cheek and stroke the inside of the cheek from top to bottom in a "C" pattern 4-5x on each side.

A Sensory Motor Approach to Feeding

EXERCISE	TARGET GROUPS	GOALS	TOOLS
Cheek Resistance	Any age Requires active movement Hypotonia Hypertonia	Cheek mobility Lip strength Lip mobility Lip rounding For feeding and speech	Gloved finger Trimmed toothette Z-Vibe® yellow preefer head with or without vibration

Place a tool inside the cheek approximately where the child would contract the cheeks for sucking (masseter muscle). Stretch the cheek outward and instruct your client to suck in or give a kiss. Repeat 4-5x on each side.

EXERCISE	TARGET GROUPS	GOALS	TOOLS
Maintaining Tongue Lateralization	Infant	Provoke and maintain tongue lateralization	Gloved finger

Place a gloved finger on the lateral border of the tongue and stroke from back to front 5x on one side and then 5x on the other side, 2 sets total.

EXERCISE	TARGET GROUPS	GOALS	TOOLS
Maintain Munch	Infant	Provoke and maintain a munch	Gloved finger or Infadent®

Place a gloved finger or Infadent on the lateral lower molar ridge. Stroke from back to front 4-5x on one side and then 4-5x on the opposite side.

EXERCISE	TARGET GROUPS	GOALS	TOOLS
Lateral Tongue Massage	Any age 1+	Elongation of the tongue and tongue lateralization	Trimmed Toothette Z-Vibe® with fine tip *(note: if there is jaw instability use Bite Block level 6 or 7 to stabilize the jaw on the opposite side of the stimulus)*

Stroke the lateral borders of the tongue from back to front 4-5x on one side and then 4-5x on the opposite side for 2 sets.

EXERCISE	TARGET GROUPS	GOALS	TOOLS
Bilateral Tongue Hugs	Any age 1+	Lingual Elongation to the lateral borders of the tongue as a pre-requisite to facilitating tongue lateralization	2 Z-Vibes® with small green square heads

Place two Z-Vibes® with small green heads on the lateral margins of the tongue. Stroke firmly from the back to the tongue tip 5x, 2 sets.

The Chewing Hierarchy

The Chewing Hierarchy was designed to sequence the oral sensory-motor skills needed for eating solid foods. It is important to remember that a pre-feeding program is always one step ahead of the feeding program. For example, if you are working on pre-feeding Chewing Hierarchy level 1 with a Chewy Tube®, or other appropriate tool, then solids have not yet been introduced. Once the child has moved to pre-feeding Chewing Hierarchy level 2 on the Chewy Tube®, or other appropriate tool, then easy-to-masticate solids can be started at Chewing Hierarchy level 1. The selection of the tool reflects the child's sensory system. If the child has no teeth, a toothette dipped in ice or a favorite puree/juice may be used. If a child is under-responsive to input, and over a year of age, a vibration tool, such as a Z-Vibe® with an appropriate tip, may be used. If a child benefits from deep pressure, a Chewy Tube® may be selected. For a child with a high fixed jaw posture, start with the yellow Chewy Tube®. If the child is in a low, poorly graded jaw posture, the red Chewy Tube® may be a better choice. The red Chewy Tube® is softer and easier to compress, and the yellow Chewy Tube® is slightly firmer. Take this into consideration if your client has reduced jaw strength. The goal is that a child can do Chewing Hierarchy level 1 for 4-5 repetitions x 2 sets, with both yellow and red Chewy Tubes®.

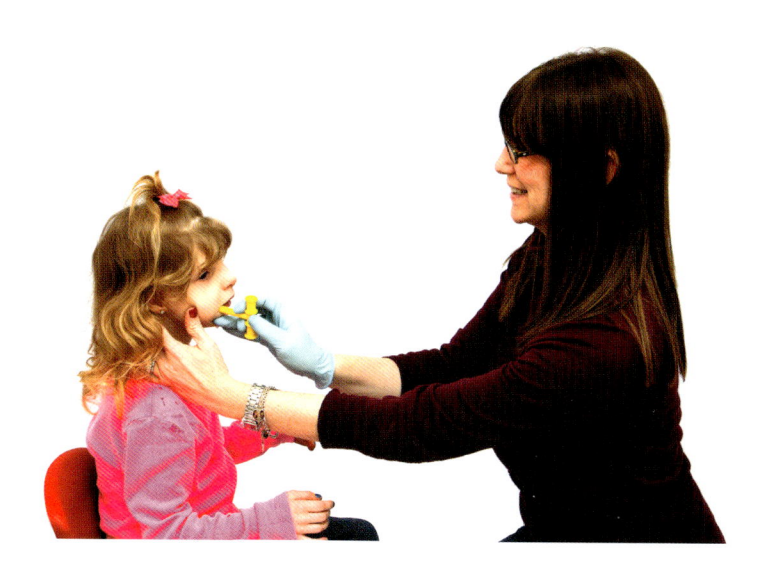

EXERCISE	TARGET GROUPS	GOALS	TOOLS
Pre-Feeding Chewing Hierarchy 1	4-6 months and up	Symmetrical chew Tongue retraction Lateral chew	Yellow and/or Red Chewy Tubes®, Z-Vibe® preefer tip (no vibration if under a year of age), Trimmed Toothette, Frozen Ice Straws*, Small green square tips, XL Bite-n-Chew head

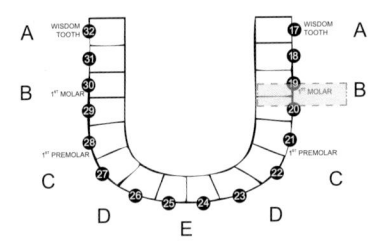

Present the tool perpendicular to the lateral molar ridge where the first molar will insert (B). Provide firm pressure into the tool to stimulate a munch chew. If necessary, support the jaw with your non dominant hand. Work toward 4-5 repetitive bites on one side and then the other. Repeat this cycle 2x.

EXERCISE	TARGET GROUPS	GOALS	TOOLS
Pre-Feeding Chewing Hierarchy 2	7-9 months and up	Tongue tip pointing Lateral chew (diagonal)	Yellow and/or Red Chewy Tubes®, Z-Vibe® preefer tip (no vibration if under a year of age), Trimmed Toothette. May use Nuk® Massager, or the XL head if rolling is needed, Frozen Ice Straws *

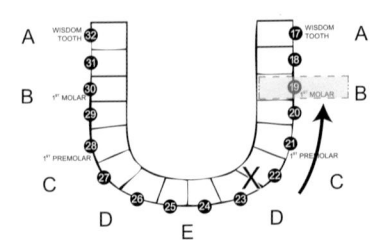

Present the tool to the lateral incisor (or where it would insert) at "D". Facilitate a bite on the lateral incisor and immediately move the tool to the location of the first molar (B) and facilitate a second bite. If the child bites on the tool and does not release it, roll the tool from the lateral incisor to the first molar. Repeat 4-5x on one side and then the other. The therapist should look for tongue lateralization from the lateral incisor (D) to the first molar (B).

A Sensory Motor Approach to Feeding

EXERCISE	TARGET GROUPS	GOALS	TOOLS
Pre-Feeding Chewing Hierarchy 3	10-12 months and up	Crossing the midline Reduce extraneous head movement secondary to unresolved rooting	2 Yellow Chewy Tubes®

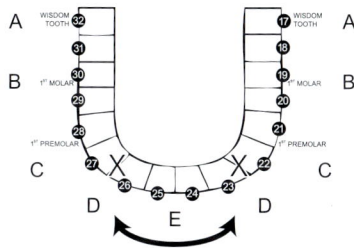

Present one yellow Chewy Tube® on the client's lateral incisor (D) and facilitate a bite. Immediately present the second Chewy Tube® on the opposite Chewy Tube® and facilitate a bite (D). Work left to right and right to left 4-5 repetitions x 2 sets. The use of two Chewy Tubes® reduces rooting and extraneous head movements, and encourages jaw stability and a dissociated bite.

EXERCISE	TARGET GROUPS	GOALS	TOOLS
Pre-Feeding Chewing Hierarchy 4	13-15 months and up	Motor plan for a rotary chew	Yellow and/or Red Chewy Tubes®, Z-Vibe® preefer tip, Trimmed Toothette, Frozen Ice Straws*, Small green square tips, XL Bite and Chew head

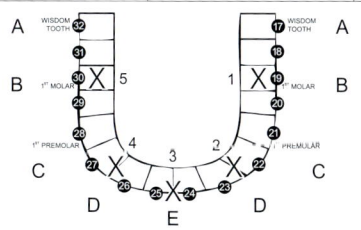

Present the tool of choice on the client's first molar (B1). Provide stability with your non dominant hand as needed. Encourage the client to do 5 small graded bites: first molar (B1), lateral incisor (D2), front central incisor (E3), lateral incisor (D4), and first molar (B5) on the opposite side. 4-5x right to left, 4-5x left to right for 2 sets. Note that everyone has a stronger side; however, if your client has significant weakness on one side you may work 2x on the weaker side as opposed to 1x on the stronger side.

*NOTE: To transition clients from pre-feeding to feeding activities, you may use an ice straw. To create this tool, place a paper clip on one end of a wide drinking straw. Use a syringe to fill the straws with a highly flavored liquid or puree such as lemonade or applesauce. Place the ice straws in a cup and freeze until firm. Use for Chewing Hierarchy levels 1, 2 and 4.

Chapter 7: A Pre-Feeding Program

Cup Drinking

Pre-requisite skills:
- Jaw stability
- Cheek contraction for sucking and swallowing
- Lip closure for swallowing liquids (upper lip should come down and forward to draw liquid in while the lower lip stabilizes the cup)
- Jaw-lip-tongue dissociation and grading
- Mobility of lateral borders of the tongue for retraction
- Mobility of the tongue tip

Pre-feeding activities to achieve these prerequisite skills:

EXERCISE	TARGET GROUPS	GOALS	TOOLS
Jiggler Roll	Any age 1+ Hypertonia Hypotonia	Upper lip mobility	Jiggler
Position the cone-shaped handle of the Jiggler horizontally under the nostrils and roll the Jiggler toward the insertion of the upper lip. Reposition the tool and repeat 4-5x.			

EXERCISE	TARGET GROUPS	GOALS	TOOLS
Mickey Mouse Ears	Any age 1+ Hypertonia Hypotonia *(if under one year use the tool without vibration)*	Upper lip mobility Lip closure	Z-Vibe® with a Mickey Mouse tip head Stabilize

A Sensory Motor Approach to Feeding

EXERCISE	TARGET GROUPS	GOALS	TOOLS
Upper Lip Strength	Any age Hypotonia Fixed upper lip Hypertonia	Upper lip mobility and strength	Gloved finger Infadent Well trimmed toothette Z-Vibe® yellow preefer head with or without vibration
Place a gloved finger or tool under the upper lip. Roll the "tool," or finger, from the corner of the lips to midline. Reposition the "tool" or finger in the opposite corner of the lips and roll to midline. Repeat this sequence 4-5x.			

EXERCISE	TARGET GROUPS	GOALS	TOOLS
Cheek Stretch	Any age Passive exercise Hypotonia Hypertonia	Cheek mobility, Lip strength, Lip mobility, Lip rounding, For feeding and speech	Infadent Yellow Z-Vibe® Tip Trimmed Toothette (nonflavored)
Place the tool in the child's cheek and stroke the inside of the cheek from top to bottom in a "C" pattern 4-5x on each side.			

EXERCISE	TARGET GROUPS	GOALS	TOOLS
Cheek resistance	Any age Requires active movement Hypotonia Hypertonia	Cheek mobility, Lip strength, Lip mobility, Lip rounding, For feeding and speech	Gloved finger Trimmed toothette Z-Vibe® yellow preefer head with or without vibration
Place a tool inside the cheek approximately where the child would contract the cheeks for sucking (masseter muscle.) Stretch the cheek outward and instruct your client to suck in or give a kiss. Repeat 4-5x on each side.			

Chapter 7: A Pre-Feeding Program

EXERCISE	TARGET GROUPS	GOALS	TOOLS
Cheek Toning/ Lip rounding	Any age Requires active movement Hypotonia Hypertonia	Cheek toning, Lip rounding, For feeding and speech	Jiggler

Provide jaw stability with your non dominant hand as needed. Place the rounded end of the Jiggler handle between your client's lips. Facilitate lip rounding with your non dominant hand. Model a "w" sound to facilitate lip protrusion. Encourage your client to imitate. Repeat 10x.

EXERCISE	TARGET GROUPS	GOALS	TOOLS
Lateral Tongue Massage	Any age 1+	Elongation of the tongue and tongue lateralization	Trimmed Toothette Z-Vibe® with fine tip *(note: if there is jaw instability use Bite Block level 6 or 7 to stabilize the jaw on the opposite side of the stimulus)*

Stroke the lateral borders of the tongue from back to front 4-5x on one side and then 4-5x on the opposite side for 2 sets.

EXERCISE	TARGET GROUPS	GOALS	TOOLS
Bilateral Tongue Hugs	Any age 1+	Lingual Elongation to the lateral borders of the tongue as a pre-requisite to facilitating tongue lateralization	2 Z-Vibes® with small green square heads

Place two Z-Vibes® with small green heads on the lateral margins of the tongue. Stroke firmly from the back to the tongue tip 5x, 2 sets.

A Sensory Motor Approach to Feeding

Straw Drinking

Pre-requisite skills:
- Lip rounding
- Cheek contraction
- Jaw stability
- Contraction through the lateral borders of the tongue for retraction
- Dissociation of jaw-lip-tongue movement
- Tongue retraction with dissociated tongue tip mobility

Pre-feeding activities to achieve these prerequisite skills:

EXERCISE	TARGET GROUPS	GOALS	TOOLS
Upper Lip Strength	Any age Hypotonia Fixed upper lip Hypertonia	Upper lip mobility and strength	Gloved finger Infadent Well trimmed toothette Z-Vibe® yellow preefer head with or without vibration
Place a gloved finger or tool under the upper lip. Roll the tool or finger, from the corner of the lips to midline. Reposition the tool or finger in the opposite corner of the lips and roll to midline. Repeat this sequence 4-5x.			

EXERCISE	TARGET GROUPS	GOALS	TOOLS
Cheek Stretch	Any age Passive exercise Hypotonia Hypertonia	Cheek mobility, Lip strength, Lip mobility, Lip rounding, For feeding and speech	Infadent Yellow Z-Vibe® Tip Trimmed Toothette (nonflavored)
Place the tool in the child's cheek and stroke the inside of the cheek from top to bottom in a "C" pattern 4-5x on each side.			

EXERCISE	TARGET GROUPS	GOALS	TOOLS
Cheek Resistance	Any age Requires active movement Hypotonia Hypertonia	Cheek mobility, Lip strength, Lip mobility, Lip rounding For feeding and speech	Gloved finger Trimmed toothette Z-Vibe® yellow preefer head with or without vibration
Place a tool inside the cheek approximately where the child would contract the cheeks for sucking (masseter muscle.) Stretch the cheek outward and instruct your client to suck in or give a kiss. Repeat 4-5x on each side.			

EXERCISE	TARGET GROUPS	GOALS	TOOLS
Vibrating kisses	Any age 1+ Hypotonia Hypertonia	Cheek toning Lip rounding	Jiggler Electric toothbrush with a small round head
Present a child-friendly vibrating toy midline on your client's lips. With your non dominant hand provide jaw support and lip rounding as needed. Model repetitive kisses using "fish lips" and encourage your client to imitate. Work up to 10 repetitive kisses.			

EXERCISE	TARGET GROUPS	GOALS	TOOLS
Cheek toning/ Lip rounding	Any age Requires active movement Hypotonia Hypertonia	Cheek toning Lip rounding For feeding and speech	Jiggler
Provide jaw stability with your non dominant hand as needed. Place the rounded end of the Jiggler handle between your client's lips. Facilitate lip rounding with your non dominant hand. Model a "w" sound to facilitate lip protrusion. Encourage your client to imitate. Repeat 10x.			

EXERCISE	TARGET GROUPS	GOALS	TOOLS
Fish Lip Pops	Any age Required active movement Hypotonia Hypertonia	Cheek mobility, Lip strength, Lip mobility, Lip rounding For feeding and speech	Infadent Yellow round Z-Vibe® Tip Trimmed Toothette (nonflavored)
Place the yellow rounded preefer tip of the Z-Vibe®, or tool of choice, between your clients's rounded lips. If necessary use your non dominant hand to support the jaw and encourage lip rounding. Encourage your client to suck in their cheeks, pucker their lips around the tool. You may use the image of a fish kiss if your client can follow this directive. Instruct the client to "pop" the tool as you remove it from their lips. Repeat 10x.			

EXERCISE	TARGET GROUPS	GOALS	TOOLS
Lateral Tongue Massage	Any age 1+	Elongation of the tongue and tongue lateralization	Trimmed Toothette Z-Vibe® with fine tip *(note: if there is jaw instability use Bite Block level 6 or 7 to stabilize the jaw on the opposite side of the stimulus)*
Stroke the lateral borders of the tongue from back to front 4-5x on one side and then 4-5x on the opposite side for 2 sets.			

EXERCISE	TARGET GROUPS	GOALS	TOOLS
Bilateral Tongue Hugs	Any age 1+	Lingual Elongation to the lateral borders of the tongue as a pre-requisite to facilitating tongue lateralization	2 Z-Vibes® with small green square heads (or blue if the client is older)
Place two Z-Vibes® with small green heads on the lateral margins of the tongue. Stroke firmly from the back to the tongue tip 5x, 2 sets.			

CONCLUSION:

The goal of a pre-feeding program is to develop the motor skills for safe, effective, nutritive feeding. A pre-feeding program is always a step ahead of a feeding program. Therapy sessions are carefully planned, secondary to a task analysis of the prerequisite skills needed for breast, bottle, spoon, cup, chewing, and straw drinking.

CHAPTER 8:
SENSORY BASED DIET SHAPING

LEADING GOALS/POINTS

Understanding the causes of a self-limited diet

Analyzing a diet profile

Evaluating the environment

Learning the process of diet shaping

Establishing a home base

Learning strategies for behavioral management in diet expansion

SELF-LIMITED DIETS ARE NOT PURELY BEHAVIORAL

As we have established, many children with self-limited diets are not choosing to eat this way. They are reacting to their deficits in sensory processing, oral sensory-motor disorders, or medical issues.

Some feeding clinics approach self-limited diets with a purely behavioral program alone. These programs seek to reinforce children for eating challenge foods with preferred foods, toys, books, or television. They do not account for the sensory and motor challenges children may be experiencing (Overland, 2011).

In addition, many children are resistant to doing therapy with food given their past negative experiences. It may then be necessary to start some children with sensory processing therapy. Prior to moving forward with diet expansion, pre-feeding activities may be used to help develop the motor skills that support feeding (Chapter 7). In addition to developing motor skills, sensory processing in the mouth can be normalized or enhanced.

For example, a child on the autism spectrum may not have muscle-based issues; however, the child's sensory system may be over-responsive. Use of a pre-feeding program with non-edibles, prior to food introduction, may help slowly shape acceptance of various food textures, temperatures, and tastes (Merkel-Walsh, 2012).

This chapter will focus on the process of diet-shaping to help expand the repertoire of foods in a client's diet.

Five-Day Baseline

In order to understand a child's diet profile, it is important to collect the necessary data and analyze that data in conjunction with information collected on the child's oral sensory-motor skill development. In order to understand taste, temperature, and texture preferences, have the caregivers fill out this form. Make sure that the parent/caregiver writes in brand names (when possible), amount consumed, and the utensils that were used (if relevant). For example, "5 pieces of Acme chicken nuggets, dipped in ketchup with his hands." (Note a reduplicable form can be found in Appendix D).

Five-Day Baseline Diet

	1	2	3	4	5
BREAKFAST					
LUNCH					
SNACK					
DINNER					
SNACK					
ADDITIONAL NOTES					

Establishing a "Home Base"

This chart should be used to establish a child's "home base." A "home base" is the taste, texture, temperature, size, and shape of food that a client prefers. Establishing a "home base" from these patterns will provide a starting point for introducing new foods.

Consider this case history

Adam is a three-year-old male with a diagnosis of Down Syndrome and Sensory Processing Disorder. His case history includes the following:

Medical History: Severe reflux, Autism Spectrum Disorder, chronic upper respiratory infections, and recurrent otitis media, and constipation.

Oral Motor and Feeding History: Adam had difficulty latching for breast feeding, secondary to oral-facial hypotonia. After the introduction of several bottle nipples, he attained adequate nutrition from a bottle using a Nuk® nipple. His mother recalls him losing a significant amount of liquid and being a noisy eater. Adam transitioned to pureed food slowly, and his parents reported that he pushed purees out of his mouth with his tongue for a long period of time. He continues to use a protrusion/retraction pattern to handle purees. Adam was referred for this evaluation because he has been unable to transition to solid foods. The introduction of solid foods resulted in significant gagging and choking followed by food refusal.

Craniofacial Observations: Adam had a high vaulted narrow palate with Class III dental malocclusion (underbite) and enlarged tonsils were noted during intraoral assessment. Mom reported that Adam is a mouth breather and snores at night.

Sensory History: Adam had difficulty tolerating face washing and brushing his teeth. He had difficulty paying attention and seemed overstimulated by auditory and visual input. He had difficulties with transitions from one activity to another. In social settings, such as supermarkets and shopping malls, he covers his eyes and/or ears and has tantrums.

Adam's Five-Day Baseline

	1	2	3	4	5
BREAKFAST	Cheerios® - dry	Cheerios® - dry	Cheerios® - dry	Cheerios® - dry	Cheerios® - dry
LUNCH	YoBaby® vanilla yogurt has to be ice cold or refuses	YoBaby® vanilla yogurt has to be ice cold or refuses	YoBaby® vanilla yogurt has to be ice cold or refuses	YoBaby® vanilla yogurt has to be ice cold or refuses	YoBaby® vanilla yogurt has to be ice cold or refuses
DINNER	Garlic hummus Pureed Chinese chicken with garlic Small pieces of ice cold pear	Stage 1 chicken with apple, add season salt (cold)	Garlic hummus Stage 1 turkey with rice, add soy sauce (cold) Frozen vanilla yogurt	Garlic hummus Pureed Chinese chicken with garlic Small pieces of ice cold pear	Pureed pasta with garlic and butter Stage 1 apple/pear with cinnamon
SNACK	Gerber® Puffs Mum Mum® Cookie Banana smoothie with Pediasure for calories	Ritz® Crackers Gerber® Puffs Banana smoothie with Pediasure for calories	Gerber® puffs Mum Mum® Cookie Banana smoothie with Pediasure for calories	Gerber® puffs Mum Mum® Cookie Banana smoothie with Pediasure for calories	Ritz® Crackers Gerber® Puffs Banana smoothie with Pediasure for calories

After the parent/caregiver completed the chart, we were able to analyze Adam's diet "home base."

PATTERN OF SENSORY CHARACTERISTICS	EXAMPLES	POSSIBLE CAUSES AND THERAPY IMPLICATIONS
Color	Adam eats all white, ivory and beige colored foods	Adam limits his diet to neutral colors which is consistent with Adam's apparent difficulty with over-stimulating environments.
Temperature	Adam eats room temperature and cold foods and liquids	Adam has low muscle-tone low tone and is under-responsive to sensory information. Cold temperatures increase sensory input and may give increased information to facilitate a swallow.
Texture	Adam is eating purees and easily chewed foods	Adam's texture preferences seem to reflect the interaction between his sensory and motor systems. He does not have the ability to break down most solid foods. He has gagged and choked on solids in the past. He eats foods that correspond to his oral sensory-motor development. The solid foods that he tolerates are easily masticated.
Taste	Adam eats salty, spicy, or sweet foods	Adam seems to need increased sensory information. This corresponds to his apparent sensory deficits. He appeared to seek increased information in the foods he chooses.
Size	Adam will only eat small pieces of easy to masticate solids such as a Cheerio®	See texture.
Shape	Client has no apparent preference.	n/a

This analysis of Adam's 5-day diet serves as a precursor for planning a program plan.

A Sensory Motor Approach to Feeding

THE ENVIRONMENT MAY SUPPORT OR NEGATE NUTRITIVE FEEDING

Evaluating the Environment

Families may report that a child eats best with a particular person or in a specific environment. It is important to assess the characteristics of the environment that support or negate nutritive feeding. As you evaluate children, it may be important to observe them in the settings in which they are most successful to determine how to modify the environment to replicate safe, nutritive feeding. It is important to take note of less successful environments. Initial questions may include:

- Does your child sit for meals or eat better if moving around the environment?
- Does your child eat better alone or with others present?
- Where does your child eat the best?
- What happens when you take your child to a restaurant?
- Does lighting, sound or climate impact your child's performance at mealtime?
- Does the style of a particular feeder impact your child's performance at mealtime?
- Does your child need to be distracted by TV, games, music, books, etc. at mealtime?

A child's program plan is developed considering the environmental characteristics. This is critical for an effective feeding plan.

Sensory State

An adequate sensory state allows an individual to be organized for feeding. For example, if your client is unable to feel hunger or thirst, tolerate the noise in the kitchen, tolerate the visual stimulus of food on their plate, or tolerate the smell of food, a complete sensory processing evaluation is warranted. Sensory supports can then be built into a client's feeding program to attain an optimum level of arousal for feeding.

The use of oral sensory input can be mapped onto the development of sensory-motor skills for feeding. These techniques are described in Chapter 9.

Diet Shaping

As you modify a diet, it is critical to make one change at a time. This helps you know what is impacting a child's behavior in relationship to food. Staying close to the "home base" and making small incremental changes in a child's diet is essential in expanding a self-limited diet.

> **MAKE ONE CHANGE AT A TIME**

The following factors can help a client expand the diet:

1. Ensure that the client is at the optimal level of arousal for feeding and that sensory supports as previously discussed are in place.

2. Place the client in a well-supported position for feeding. If the client has low muscle tone, the seating position should ensure that the hips and knees are at a 90-degree angle and the feet are grounded. The feet should be grounded and the head should be in neutral flexion.

3. Using the activities in Chapter 7, develop the motor skills to support feeding.

4. Stay close to the client's "home base," and make small incremental changes in the client's diet.

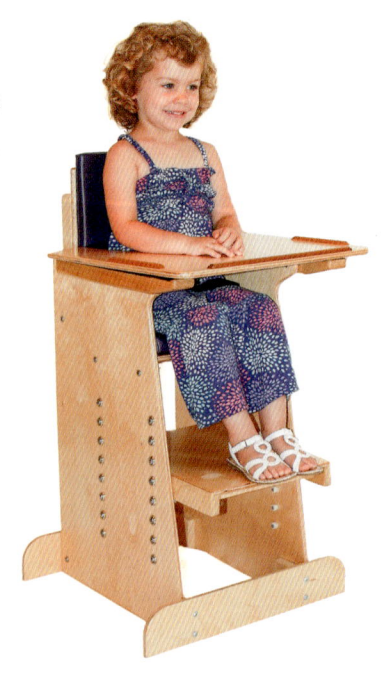

5. Make only one change at a time, so that it is clear what is impacting the client's behavior in relation to food.

6. Consider that changing temperature and taste primarily impacts a client's sensory system.

7. Do not change texture until the client has the sensory-motor skills to support the new texture.

8. Consider the size of the bolus. The bolus must be big enough to feel and small enough to handle safely.

9. Consider shape and placement of the bolus. Where you place food in the mouth will impact the sensory-motor skills. Bolus shape is discussed in Chapter 9.

10. Hiding foods within another texture is counterproductive, i.e., a parent hides peas in mashed potatoes, because the child loves mashed potatoes. This may cause the child to refuse the preferred item, and distrust previously accepted food items. This also creates a mixed texture which requires different motor skills, and could result in gagging, choking, or vomiting.

Consider this case study that included diet shaping

In a 5-day baseline diet, it was noted that a 6-year old boy with a primary diagnosis of Autism Spectrum Disorder ate a great deal of high-taste crunchy foods, but was not eating enough protein or fresh produce. Typical foods consumed were: Cheetos®, Doritos®, sugary dry cereals, french fries, chicken nuggets, potato chips, and sour cream and onion flavored chips and crackers. Everything was basically room temperature. The client would only eat chicken nuggets if they were fresh from McDonald's®, and they could not be reheated or get too cold. If foods touched one another the child would refuse to eat them. The child tended to overstuff and pocket food, and used his fingers to move bolus across the midline. He ate better at school with peer models, but would still not deviate from his self-limited diet. The boy also rocked his body while eating. His mother reported he liked ketchup and, on occasion, he would eat it with a spoon. He also liked to dunk most foods in ketchup. "Home Base": crunchy, room temperature, salty, high-taste foods.

Environment: seeks movement while eating, and benefits from peer models.

Sensory State: seeks increased input from foods, such as dipping in ketchup. Potential visual sensitivity (i.e., cannot tolerate foods touching each other or more than one food on his plate at a time). Seeks movement while eating, such as rocking. This was observed secondary to reduced ability to masticate and motor plan the sequence of placing/collecting a bolus and swallowing.

Pre-feeding program: A plan was designed to develop the motor skills to support safe, nutritive feeding.

Diet Shaping

START	PHASE 1	PHASE 2	PHASE 3	PHASE 4
Chicken nuggets	Slightly warm nugget	Serve the nuggets with a dip of half ketchup/half mayo to add new taste + fat from egg protein	Try a new brand of chicken nugget at the same temperature with the same dip	Try fish sticks, or chicken with homemade crunchy breading such as panko
Sour cream and onion chips	Try the same chips with a sour cream and onion dip made with greek yogurt for protein	Try new chips with similar visual characteristics or crackers with same dip	Try new crunchy snacks with various dips such as hummus	Introduce dehydrated vegetables such as yucca chips, green beans and "Veggie Chips" with the same dips
French fries	Try french fries with seasoned salt	Change the texture of the fries by making home-made oven fries, a healthier alternative	Try sweet potato fries baked the same way as the new oven fry	Slice zucchini, eggplant and carrot into thin strips. Coat with crunchy breading and fry.

Additional Examples

Here are examples on how to change foods one element at a time. Note that these changes are specific to an individual child. Some children may need even smaller changes:

START FOOD	ELEMENT OF CHANGE	NEW FOOD
Chicken Nuggets	Taste	Add seasoned salt to batter
Apple	Taste	Try pear – firm
Apple sauce	Temperature*	Place in freezer for 10 minutes before therapy
Cheerios®	Taste	Try Apple Cinnamon variety
French Fries	Texture	Place in microwave and then allow to cool for chewiness
Mac and Cheese	Taste	Add a new cheese to the recipe
Pasta with Butter	Taste	Add Parmesan cheese
Pasta with Red Sauce	Texture	Cook the pasta extra firm (al dente)
Boiled hot dog - no bun	Texture	Broil the hot dog
Baby Food - Apricot	Texture	Thicken with rice cereal
Grapes	Temperature*	Freeze the grapes

Reducing temperature or placing food in the freezer also alters the texture as it makes foods more dense

Behavior Strategies

ABA IS A USEFUL STRATEGY

While this book focuses primarily on sensory-motor feeding disorders and techniques, the following is a brief outline of Applied Behavioral Analysis (ABA) techniques that are useful in supporting feeding therapy.

While most children with self-limited diets have sensory and/or motor issues, behavioral issues may be secondary. It is rare that a feeding disorder is purely behavioral; however, it does occur. In cases where feeding issues have become behavioral (e.g., for some clients with Autism Spectrum Disorder), the principles of Applied Behavioral Analysis (ABA) are useful in feeding therapy (Roche et al, 2011). ABA is a teaching technique that has positive empirical research for teaching children with autism; therefore, the principles of ABA teaching can be very valuable when implementing feeding programs (McEachin et al., 1993; Merkel-Walsh, 2012).

Children with behavioral issues may present in several ways. Picture the low tone child who typically has an open mouth posture at rest. When a food with which they are uncomfortable comes near that child's mouth, he/she immediately exhibits tight, fixed-lip closure and moves away from the bolus. This child is exhibiting a behavior, but has a clear oral sensory-motor response (fixing).

Picture another child with an impaired sensory system who screams uncontrollably at the sight of a nonpreferred food. This child may lash out physically and injure himself or the feeder when a new food is presented.

For children who exhibit these types of behaviors and are already receiving ABA therapy, an ABC format can be used in feeding sessions analyzing: Antecedent, Behavior, and Consequence. Negative reinforcement or inappropriate positive reinforcement can inadvertently contribute to a feeding disorder. Here are some examples:

ANTECEDENT	BEHAVIOR	CONSEQUENCE
Parent presents food	Child spits out food	Parent yells at child (negative reinforcement)
Parent presents food	Child eats food	Parent gives child a lollipop (positive reinforcement)
Parent presents food	Child hits parent	Parent ignores behavior and represents food (ignoring/extinction)
Parent presents food	Child vomits	Parent cleans up child and does not try to feed again (inadvertent reinforcement of an undesirable behavior)

The way in which we respond to a behavior can reinforce a child either positively or negatively. Parents, without knowing it, sometimes inadvertently reinforce nonproductive feeding patterns that need to be corrected.

In feeding sessions, it is critical that positive responses are reinforced and that negative responses are ignored, when possible, since we understand that many feeding disorders come from sensory-motor problems. We need to address feeding disorders as a complex manifestation of behavior and sensory-motor challenges (Roche et al., 2011).

Examples of Behavioral Supports

Token boards, or sequencing boards, are useful as teaching tools. A token board rewards the client for a target behavior. The client is usually working for a target reward such as watching a DVD, using an electronic device, or playing with a toy. Here is an example of a token board used with a 5-year-old child:

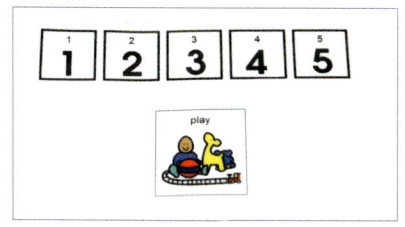

The child is required to take five bites of a target food before earning a reward. With this particular board, the cubes of food were placed on the numbers, so the child had concrete visual stimuli.

Using this next token board, the child earned a token for every three bites of food. After 15 bites, he earned the opportunity to put together a puzzle:

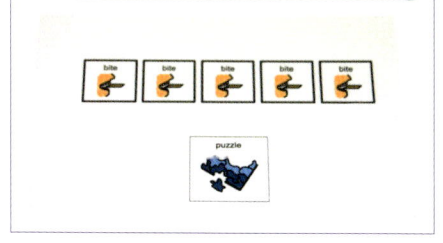

Sequencing boards can also help children understand the rhythm of feedings such as the bite, chew, and swallow sequence. Here is a sequencing board that highlights the steps of feeding (e.g., bite, chew, swallow/food goes in the belly, take a drink) using Mayer-Johnsons's Picture Communication Symbols:

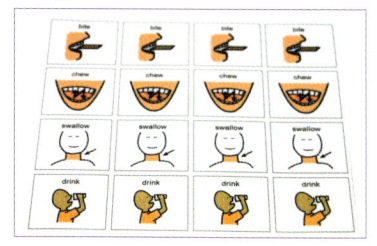

ABA therapy allows parents, therapists, and others to break down tasks into achievable short-term objectives (STO). When we combine this with sensory-motor goals we can successively approximate steps moving toward the long-term goal of diet expansion. It is important to remember that ABA and other forms of behavior modification need to be combined with the implementation of sensory-motor goals (Roche et al., 2011). A child may need to become accustomed to the sight, the smell, and the feel of a food, prior to managing and swallowing it. While the therapist is targeting the sensory-motor feeding techniques found in Chapter 9, the therapist can be simultaneously helping the child become accustomed to new foods via an ABA or other behavior modification approach. A sequential hierarchy is often recommended to introduce a new food. The Sequential Oral Sensory (SOS) approach is one program that systematically introduces foods (Toomey & Sundseth, 2011). For example the child will be asked to:

1. Look at the food
2. Touch the food
3. Tolerate the food near the mouth
4. Kiss the food
5. Taste the food
6. Chew the food
7. Swallow the food

CONCLUSION:

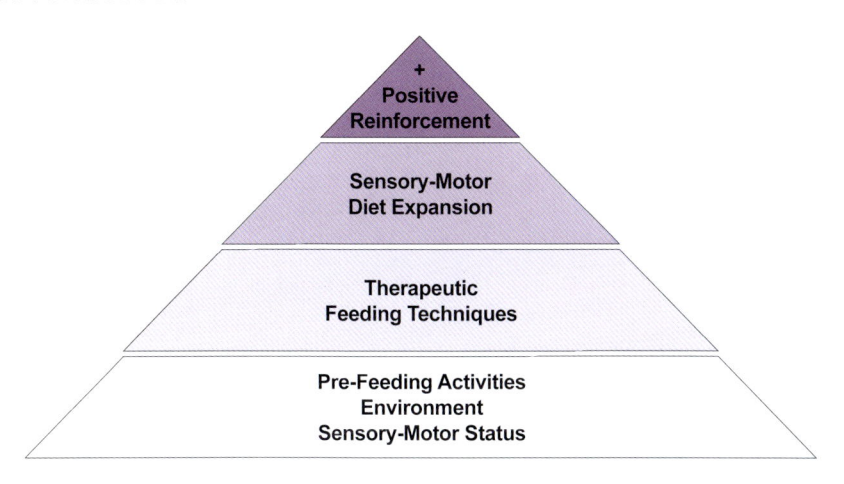

```
            +
         Positive
       Reinforcement

       Sensory-Motor
       Diet Expansion

       Therapeutic
      Feeding Techniques

    Pre-Feeding Activities
         Environment
      Sensory-Motor Status
```

Following the analysis of a five-day baseline the clinician can establish the client's "home base." In conjunction with a sensory-motor approach and appropriate behavior management, a feeding program for sensory-motor diet expansion can be implemented. The therapist can start with the sensory-motor status and then build a program from the ground up, considering: the environment, selected pre-feeding activities (Chapter 7), therapeutic feeding activities (Chapter 9), and diet expansion. Each level of this pyramid should be reinforced positively through behavior modification techniques for optimum progress levels.

CHAPTER 9:
THERAPEUTIC FEEDING

LEADING GOALS/POINTS

Learning to plan a feeding program

Understanding the importance of positioning, food choices, sensory-motor diet shaping, utensils, food placement and supports

Task analysis of the oral motor skills required for safe and effective nutritive feeding

The goal of a therapeutic feeding program is to develop the sensory-motor skills for safe, effective, nutritive feeding. Remember that your pre-feeding program is always a step ahead of your feeding program (Overland, 2011). For example, if your client is ready to work on cup drinking, you have already worked on the pre-feeding skills needed, including: lip closure, cheek contraction, and tongue retraction as described in Chapter 7.

Some considerations before starting a Therapeutic Feeding Program:
- A pre-feeding program has been initiated
- The child is at his/her optimal state of arousal
- An Occupational Therapist has been consulted regarding sensory processing
- A Physical Therapist has been consulted regarding positioning
- A nutritionist has been consulted regarding caloric goals
- Your client's physician has been consulted regarding medical issues

Planning a Program

The following hierarchy can be used to plan a therapeutic feeding program:

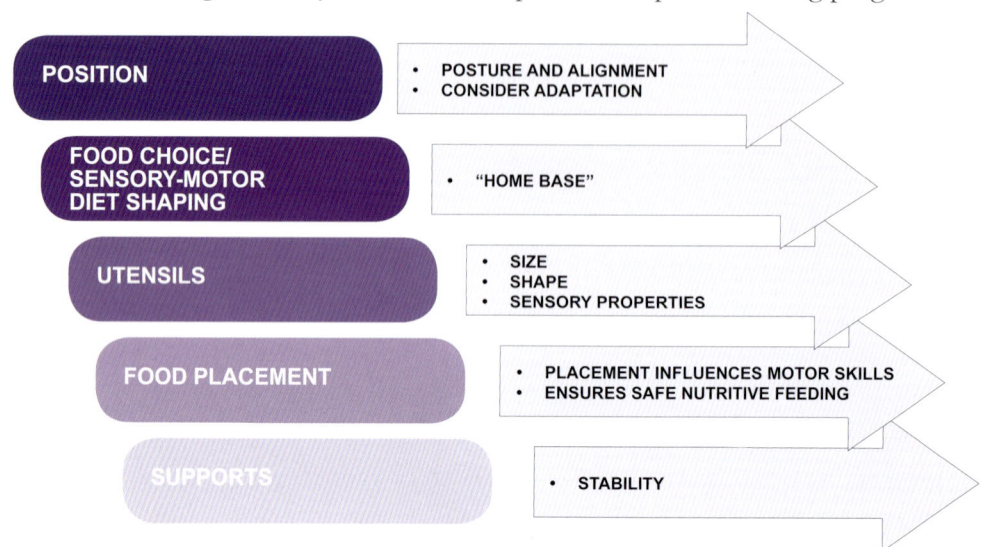

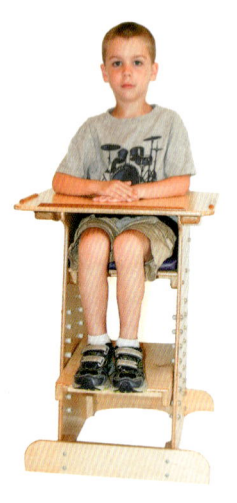

POSITION	• POSTURE AND ALIGNMENT • CONSIDER ADAPTATION
FOOD CHOICE/ SENSORY-MOTOR DIET SHAPING	• "HOME BASE"
UTENSILS	• SIZE • SHAPE • SENSORY PROPERTIES
FOOD PLACEMENT	• PLACEMENT INFLUENCES MOTOR SKILLS • ENSURES SAFE NUTRITIVE FEEDING
SUPPORTS	• STABILITY

1. Position — Postural control and alignment are the foundation for all motor activities. Clients with compromised postural systems often require assisted stability in order to be

> **WHAT YOU SEE IN THE BODY IS WHAT YOU GET IN THE MOUTH**

successful oral feeders. One optimal position is when the trunk is aligned and stabilized, the head is aligned in neutral flexion, the hands are at midline, the hips are at a 90-degree angle, the knees are at a 90-degree angle, and the feet are grounded. Depending upon your client's postural restrictions and muscle tone, adaptations may need to be made. It is also important for the feeder to be at eye level with the child, to ensure posture and alignment in the head and neck. You may need to consult with the client's physical and/or occupational therapist for positioning recommendations.

2. Food Choice/Sensory-Motor Diet Shaping —
Choose foods based on your client's sensory and motor skills as outlined in Chapter 8. Remember to stay close to your client's "home base" and

make one change at a time.

3. Utensils — The size, shape, and sensory properties of the utensils will influence your clients' sensory-motor skills. For example, sterling silver spoons dipped in ice maintain the cold for some clients that benefit from increased sensory information. Vibrating spoons may increase muscle firing and facilitate lip closure in some children. Coated spoons may protect client's teeth (e.g., those who have drop seizures during meals). Flat-bowled spoons can be used to facilitate lip closure.

> **PLACEMENT OF THE FOOD INFLUENCES HOW THE FOOD IS HANDLED**

4. Food Placement — Where you put food in the mouth influences the sensory-motor skills you use to handle the food. Imagine biting a Cheeto® with your front central incisors. Notice how your tongue moves forward to meet the bolus. Now bite the Cheeto®, which you have placed perpendicular to your first molar. Notice how your tongue is retracted and lateralized. If you do not have the ability to move food to the molar ridge for mastication, side placement may be used. Side placement surpasses the need to move the bolus using the tongue tip and the lateral borders of the tongue. Where we place food can help develop oral sensory-motor skills, ensure safe nutritive feeding, and compensate for motor weaknesses.

5. Supports — For many clients, physical supports provide stability so they can access the motor skills for feeding. Clients may need support while they learn the motor plan for feeding. Clients who have compromised neuromotor systems may always need physical support. Two effective supports are:

- a. **"V" support for the head, jaw and lips:** As you position your hip next to your client's shoulder, use your forearm to support the client's head and a "v" finger position (your middle finger under the client's jaw and pointer under the client's lower lip).

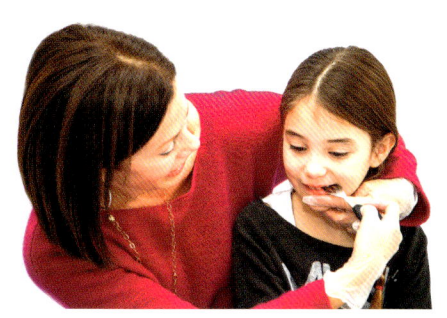

Chapter 9: Therapeutic Feeding

b. **"C" support for jaw/lip:** The pointer finger is under the jaw, while the thumb is under the lower lip for support (photo). Jaw support for stability allows for cheek and lip mobility. The cheeks help stabilize the bolus during chewing, and the lips maintain the bolus intra-orally.

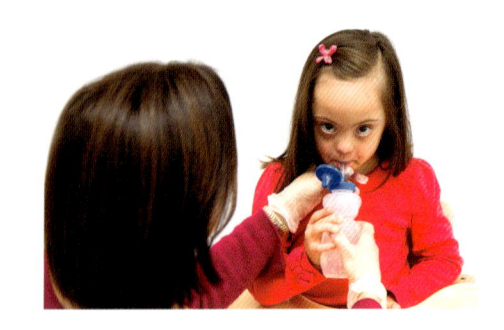

Task Analysis

In consideration of the feeding hierarchy, this chapter provides task analysis for developing feeding programs for: breast, bottle, spoon, solids, cup, and straw.

Breast Feeding

Breast feeding is almost always the preferred mode of nutrition for newborn babies. Breast-fed babies receive important antibodies from mothers' milk. Breast feeding has many benefits such as reducing food allergies, and supporting brain development (Bahr, 2010). There are several books that specifically focus on breast feeding, such as Catherine Watson-Genna's book *Supporting Sucking Skills in Breastfeeding Infants*.

Prerequisite Skills: The full-term infant is born with hard-wired synergies called oral reflexes, as described in Chapter 2. The infant's softly cupped tongue supports the nipple. A seal is formed between the tongue and the hard palate. The fatty sucking pads provide support. The tongue and the lips help to form a latch on the nipple. There is a non-dissociated jaw-tongue-cheek-lip movement which is rhythmic. Excursions of the jaw should be small and graded. (Review "Suck" definition in Chapter 2).

Clinical Suggestions

In addition to the considerations found in the chart below, it will be important that the mother's neck and back are supported and protected during feedings (Bahr, 2010). The mother needs to be comfortable as well, or this will be communicated to her baby.

POSITION

Position is contingent upon the size and shape of the mom's breasts and the infant's motor skills. The head must be maintained at a 45 to 90-degree angle.

1. A football hold allows you to support the infant's body under your arm.

2. A traditional hold may incorporate the use of a Boppy® or My Brest Friend® to support the mom's arm and the infant's body.

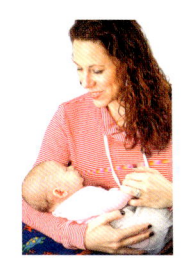

3. A side lying position for premature infants for both breast and bottle feeding. Side lying decreases the transit time, and may prevent pharyngeal pooling for infants who are having difficulty coordinating suck, swallow, breathe.

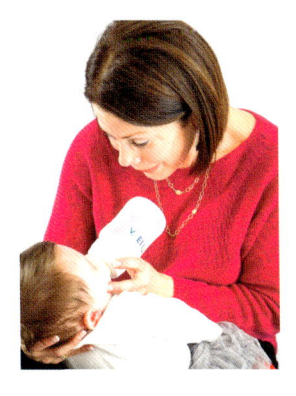

POSITION

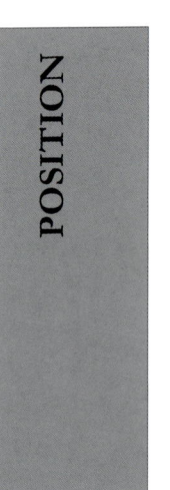

4. In Semi-Prone feeding the mother's body is reclined and semi prone, supported with pillows. The baby is positioned diagonally or horizontally on mother's body. This allows the baby to more effectively regulate milk flow and may help prevent reflux.

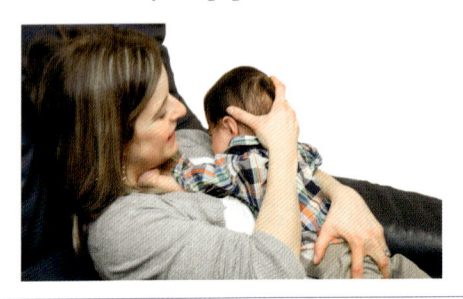

FOODS

1. If a mother is breast feeding, and the infant has allergies/sensitivities or food intolerances, the mother may go on an elimination diet. This is when the mother removes potentially allergenic foods from her diet and gradually reintroduces foods, charting the infant's reaction.

2. If latching is difficult even with therapeutic supports, breast milk may be pumped and fed via bottle feeding (see Bottle Feeding in the next segment of this chapter).

UTENSILS

1. A breast shield can be used if a mother has inverted or small nipples. The shield is used to help elongate the nipple if a) inverted; b) small; or c) the infant has difficulty latching. A breast shield can reduce the flow of milk if a letdown is too rapid for the infant to handle.

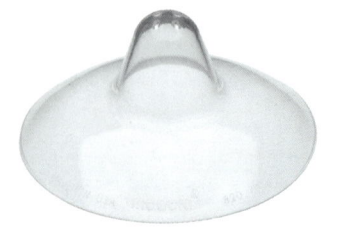

UTENSILS

2. Medela's Supplemental Nursing System® can be filled with additional breast milk allowing the infant to suck from the nipple and the supplemental nursing tube simultaneously. The system allows for additional calories with a minimal amount of work. This is helpful when the infant has a weak suck.

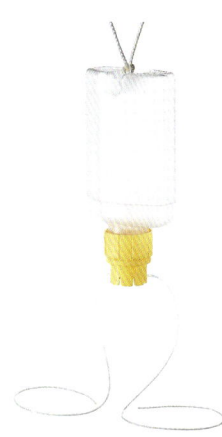

3. A syringe with a tube can be used for infants who do not have a productive suck, to supplement breast feeding, or to provide nutritive feeding as you work on the sensory-motor skills used in breast feeding.

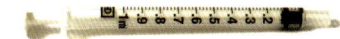

4. Boppy® pillow, Lycra breast feeding sling, and My Brest Friend® are items that can assist with positioning.

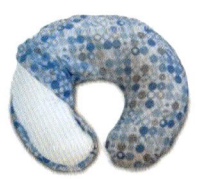

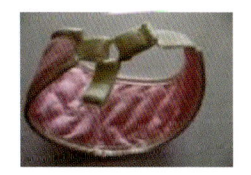

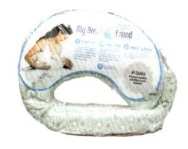

Boppy® Pillow   Breast Sling   My Brest Friend®

Bottle Feeding

Bottle feeding is an acceptable option for infants who are not successful on the breast, or if the mother has a medical condition that prevents breast feeding. It should be noted that Electro Myographic Studies (EMG) have shown differences between the muscle activation for breast versus bottle feeding, which may be secondary to flow rate (Genna, 2012).

Prerequisite Skills: The full-term infant is born with hard-wired synergies called oral reflexes, as described in Chapter 2. The infant's softly cupped tongue supports the nipple. A seal is formed between the tongue and the hard palate. The fatty sucking pads provide lateral support. The tongue and the lips help to form a latch on the nipple. In bottle feeding there is more activation of the buccinators and obicularis oris muscles than in breast feeding (Genna, 2012). There is a non-dissociated jaw-tongue-cheek-lip movement that is rhythmic and wave-like. In bottle feeding there should be equal protrusion–retraction during tongue movement to the lower gum. The tongue should not protrude outside of the mouth, nor should it be "humped."

Clinical Suggestions

It will be important to use the environment or supports to ensure that the mother's neck and back are protected during feedings. See breast feeding section for suggestions.

POSITION

1. Caretaker is seated on a bed, couch, or chair with an ottoman. Knees are bent, and the infant is positioned on the knees/upper legs facing the feeder, with the infant's head on the feeder's knees. The infant's body is supported by the upper legs on the feeder.

2. A traditional hold can be used, with the feeder's arm supported by the arm of the chair, pillow, or a Boppy® Pillow. The infant's head should be maintained at a 45 to 90-degree angle.

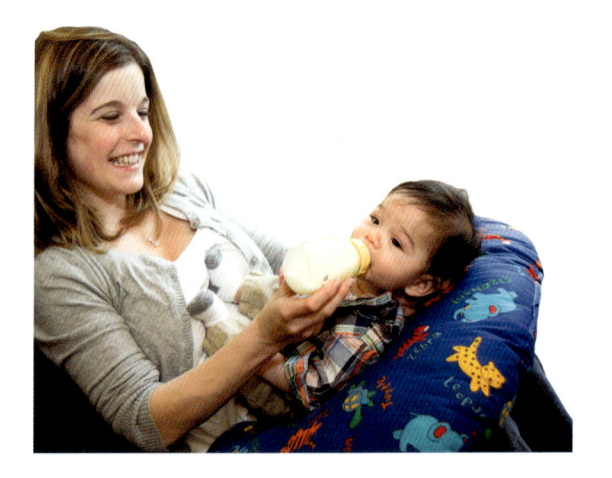

FOODS

Breast milk can be pumped and presented in a bottle. If this is not possible, there are many formula options:

- Premature Formulas
- Cow Milk Based
- Lactose Free
- Soy Based
- Hydrolyzed Whey
- Hydrolyzed Casein
- Amino Acid Based
- Pre-Thickened Formulas for GERD
- Medically Based/High Calorie Formulas
- Goat's Milk/Rice Milk (these are not complete nutritional substances and need to be supplemented)

Note: Traditional infant formulas are approximately 20 calories per ounce. High-calorie formulas can provide up to 30 calories per ounce. The water to powder ratio can be manipulated to concentrate the formula and increase calorie content for infants who fatigue easily. For infants with GERD, concentration of the formula is preferred, as opposed to thickening the formula with rice cereal or a commercial thickener (Huang et al., 2002). Simply Thick® has been linked to gasterointestinal issues in premature infants (Shrader & Associates, 2011). Recently, there have been reports that any commercial thickener is questionable for any child under a year of age.

UTENSILS

1. Recommended bottles have a vent system (e.g., Born Free®, Dr. Brown's®, Advent®), a bag system (such as Playtex Nurser®) or a crooked neck (i.e. Playtex Ventaire®) to decrease intake of air and allow an infant to be fed in an upright position, with the ears higher than the mouth.

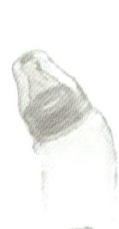

   CROOKED NECK VARIETY

2. Nipple characteristics are important. Choose a nipple that fits the size and shape of the infant's mouth. There are many manufacturers to choose from. Focus on the characteristics of the nipple. The nipple should shape the bowl of the tongue. If the nipple is too big, you may see tongue protrusion past the lower lip, or gagging. The base of the nipple should also be considered. Infants who are losing liquid may benefit from a wider base.

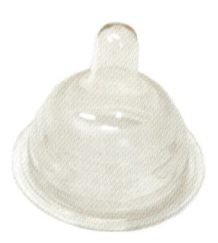

   WIDE BASED   NARROW BASED

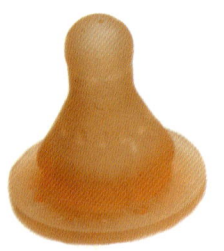

UTENSILS

3. Silicone nipples are firmer than traditional nipples. If a baby is compressing a nipple and getting too much air, you may need a firmer nipple. In contrast, if a baby is struggling to draw the liquid, you may need a softer nipple.

   NON-LATEX SOFT   SILICONE FIRM

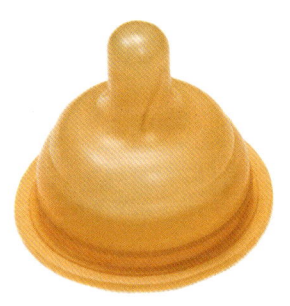

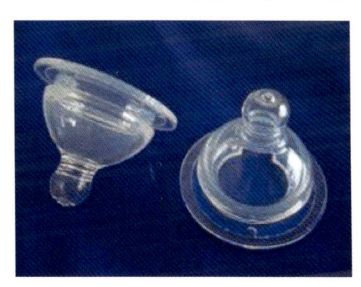

4. The shape and size of the teat should be considered. Longer teats may gag infants who have small mouths. Rounded teats may support tongue cupping, while flat teats may flatten and retract the tongue and contribute to the use of a compression release pattern to draw liquid.

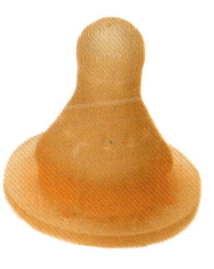

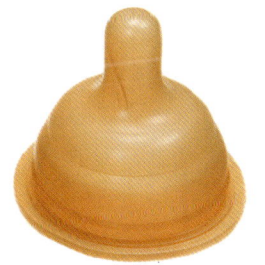

   SHORT TEAT   LONG TEAT

UTENSILS

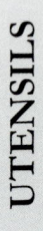

5. For infants with cleft lips and/or palates, the Haberman Feeder from Medela® can help to facilitate a latch. Pigeon nipples are another option.

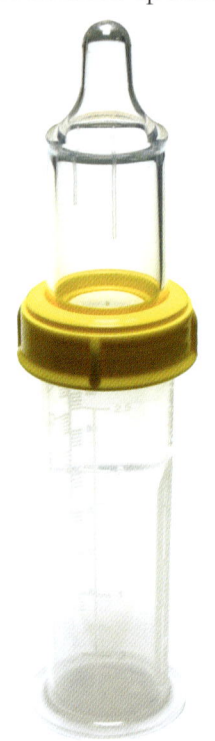

6. Flow: Choose a flow that allows an infant to coordinate suck, swallow, and breathe. If the flow is too fast, you may see pooling of formula or hear gasping, gulping or yelping sounds. If the flow is too slow, the infant may have difficulty drawing liquid and may tire quickly.

A Sensory Motor Approach to Feeding

PLACEMENT

Midline positioning of the nipple into the infant's mouth.

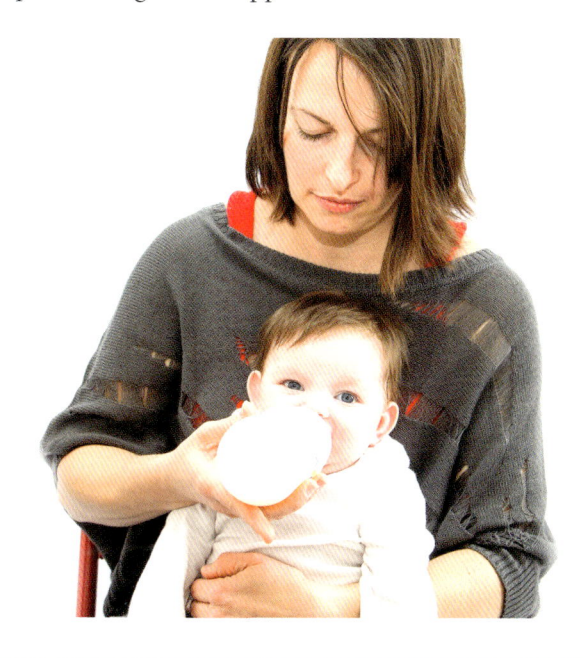

SUPPORT

1. Place the middle finger under the jaw, with the thumb and pointer finger on each check. Slowly and rhythmically rock your hand forward to the rhythm of the suck-swallow (1 beat per second).

2. Music may facilitate an infant's development of a rhythmic suck-swallow-breathe synchrony.

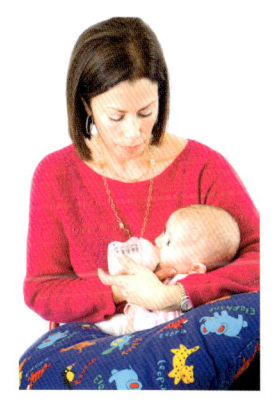

3. The feeder may need to pace the infant if respiration is compromised. Nipple can be removed or the bottle can be tilted to stop the flow of liquid.

4. Feeding schedules can be manipulated if the infant takes only small amounts of liquid at a time. Infants with reflux can be given small quantities with more frequent feedings, if the child's pediatrician agrees.

Spoon

Current medical practice usually suggests beginning spoon feeding at approximately 6 months of age, secondary to the growing number of children who have food allergies or intolerances. Typically developing infants should have head control before starting spoon feeding. Children with neuro-motor or muscle tone issues may need to have postural supports.

Prerequisite Skills: Sensory-motor skills that support spoon feeding include the ability to grade the jaw and stabilize in a mid-jaw position as the spoon enters the oral cavity. The upper lip comes forward and down to remove the food from the spoon, and the lower lip rolls inward slightly to stabilize the spoon. There is also slight tongue bowling/cupping, contraction through the lateral borders of the tongue, tongue tip elevation, tongue retraction, and cheek contraction for oral transport of the bolus.

Clinical Suggestions

- If your client is an independent eater, take turns during meal or snack time so that you are maintaining independence while facilitating improved sensory-motor skills.

- You may need to start therapeutic feeding programs slowly. If the techniques make mealtime longer, begin with 4-5 repetitions of therapeutic feeding at each meal. Encourage caregivers to continue with nutritive feedings after therapeutic feeding tasks to support optimum nutrition.

- As a client accommodates, slowly increase the repetitions at each meal by one trial at a time.

- For all feeding positions, the feeder should be eye level or below the child to ensure the maintenance of an appropriate head position.

POSITION

1. For infants, a car seat with the handle rolled as far back as possible may be used. A thick book placed under the handle will insure that the infant's head position is at a 60 to 90-degree angle. You might use the smallest Boppy® pillow to provide head support. You can also feed the child in an infant bouncy seat, fitted with head support. (Note: chair should be static, not bouncing). The Snuggin Go® supporting positioners can also be used in a car seat or infant chair for increased postural stability.

2. For infants with neuro-motor issues, a Tumble Form® chair or Special Tomato® may allow for appropriate head support, lateral support, and trunk support.

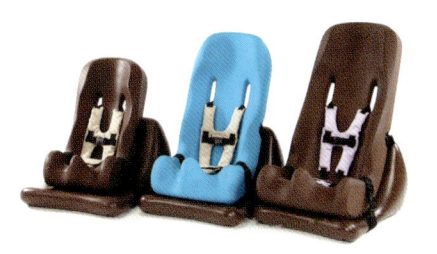

3. As infants get older, a high chair with a narrow seat, high back, pummel, foot support, and a good hip strap is recommended. Many commercial highchairs have tilting backs, which are contraindicated for children with feeding disorders. Tray position should allow for bent elbows to be supported. Booster seats should have similar characteristics.

SVAN® HIGH CHAIR

Chapter 9: Therapeutic Feeding

POSITION

FISHER PRICE® BOOSTER SEAT

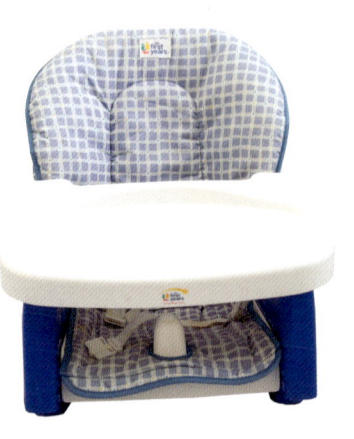

HEIGHT RIGHT BY SPECIAL TOMATO®

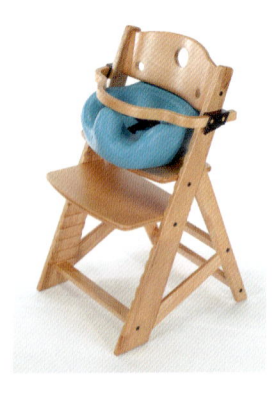

4. For toddlers who need more support, a Rifton® offers many options, including foot support, hip straps, high backs, a movable back, pummels, and well placed trays.

RIFTON® CHAIR

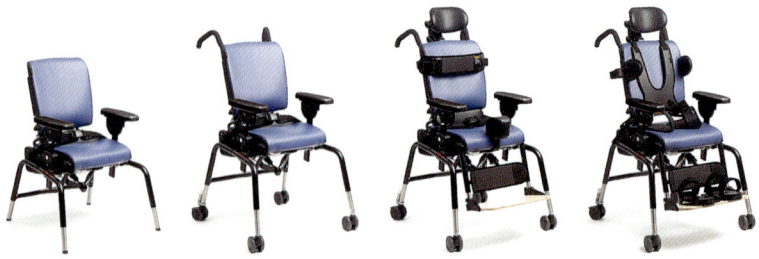

POSITION

5. Adaptive feeding chairs or wheelchairs provide stability for feeding.

    TALKTOOLS® CHAIR

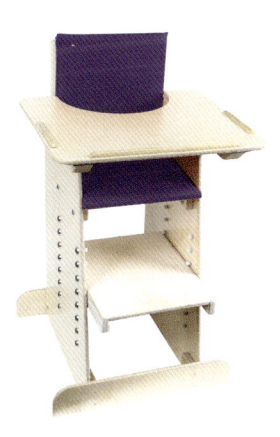

6. For some clients with significant neuromotor issues, positioning in a stander or side lyer may be appropriate during feeding.

7. Children and adults who can sit independently should be positioned in chairs that support the hips and knees in a 90- degree angle and with feet grounded. For low tone clients who fall into a posterior pelvic tilt, a wedge may be helpful.

FOODS

1. Infants:
    - At approximately 6 months of age, introduce foods one at a time.

    - Wait 4-5 days between the introductions of each new food. Watch for allergic reactions or food sensitivities, which may include: respiratory issues, rashes, vomiting, changes in bowels, behavioral changes (FAAN, 2012).

    - Initially, offer approximately one tablespoon of each new food (slowly increase).

    - Many pediatricians recommend starting babies on rice cereal, progressing to oatmeal and mixed cereals, then adding low allergy/sensitivity fruits such as applesauce, pears, then vegetables, and finally meats. However, there is some debate over whether to begin with rice and grains, given the large number of allergies to gluten (FAAN, 2012). There is also a concern about arsenic in rice cereal. An alternative approach is to begin with vegetables that are high in iron (sweet potato, carrot, broccoli, zucchini, squash), and then progress to foods that are high in zinc (banana, pears, apricots). For this approach, rice cereal is added to the diet at about nine months of age, but other grains and dairy are not introduced until well over a year (D. Wilson, personal communication, August 17, 2012).

    - Many pediatricians recommend not offering honey, egg whites, shellfish, nut products (especially peanuts), and citrus until closer to two years of age. If dairy allergies are noted in infancy, some gastroenterologists and allergists recommend a soy, dairy, nut, egg, and gluten free diet until 12-18 months of age.

FOODS

- Cultural differences influence how foods are introduced. In some cultures, babies go from breast to solids (e.g., baby-led weaning) introduced from mom's plate (mashed up, chewed up), rather than progressing to purees and then solids.

2. As foods are introduced, take into account your client's sensory system. If the child was breast fed, he/she had the taste of a variety of foods that mom was eating, so bland pureed baby food may be unappealing. Think about pureeing family foods and changing the temperature or adding additional taste to pureed foods. Blenders, such as the Baby Cook® or the Vitamix® aid in taking food from the table to a Stage 1 consistency.

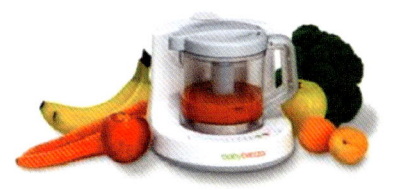

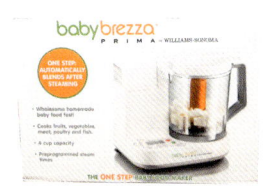

3. For clients with neuromotor issues who are on long-term pureed diets, make sure the taste of the food agrees with their sensory systems and the variety of foods presented is age appropriate. Note: blenders are also helpful in preparing foods for those individuals who are on enteral feedings and are transitioning to oral feeds. Putting real blended table foods into the enteral tubes prepares the digestive system for oral feeding (Morris & Klein, 2000).

UTENSILS

Consider the shape, size and sensory properties of spoons:

1. Flat bowled spoons and spoons with slightly elongated bowls support therapeutic spoon feeding.

    MAROON SPOONS

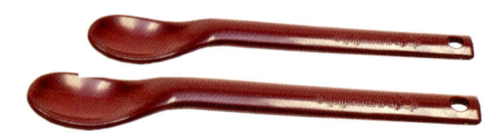

    BECKMAN® E-Z SPOONS

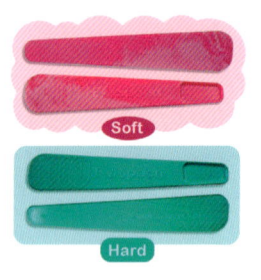

2. Deep spoons are not recommended as they encourage stabilizing with the front central incisors. Most regular teaspoons and plastic spoons have bowls that are too deep for therapeutic feeding.

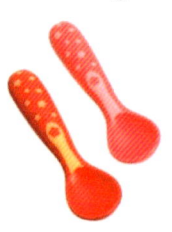

3. Coated spoons are often used with clients who have seizures. They can also be useful for clients who have sensitive teeth. However, coated spoons may hold the smell and taste of food, even after they are washed. If a child has sensory issues this may not be advisable.

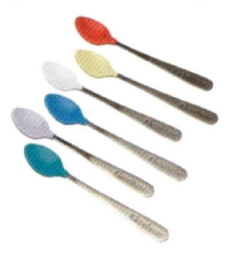

A Sensory Motor Approach to Feeding

UTENSILS

4. If a client needs increased sensory input, consider using a sterling silver spoon dipped in ice chips (it will hold the cold) or a vibrating spoon.

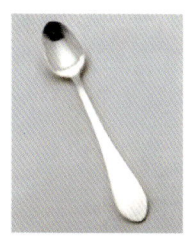

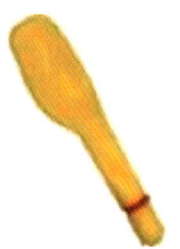

5. If a child has a retracted lower lip, a spoon with a textured bottom may be considered.

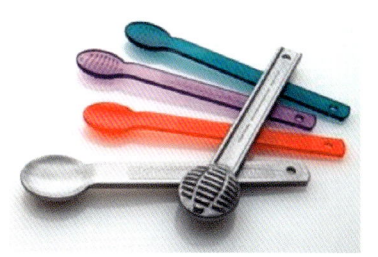

PLACEMENT

1. In order to facilitate lip closure and tongue retraction, present the spoon sideways contacting the corners of the lips.

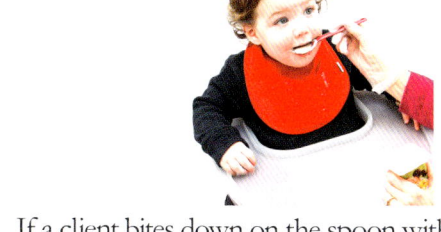

2. If a client bites down on the spoon with his/her front central incisors, tilt the spoon upward toward the upper lip.

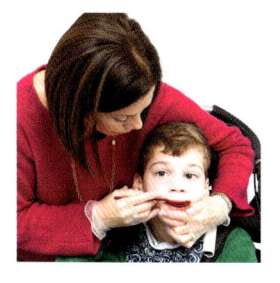

PLACEMENT

3. If a client closes his/her lips to clear the spoon and then uses a lingual protrusion to facilitate oral transport, consider a rapid repetitive technique. With this technique, the client removes half of the bolus off the spoon, then you immediately rotate the wrist and present the spoon handle contacting the opposite corner of the lip. You are facilitating the motor plan for lip closure/tongue retraction.

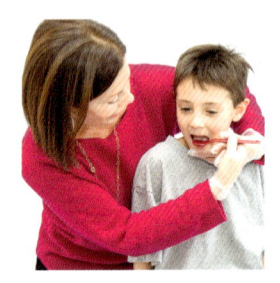

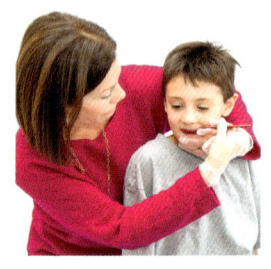

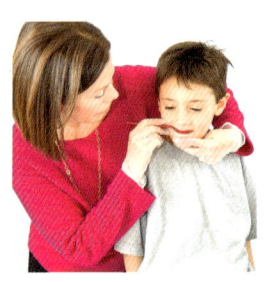

4. In general, pushing against the tongue is contraindicated to facilitate tongue retraction, particularly if the child has any form of a tongue thrust. Pushing against the tongue generally results in bulging or protrusion. However, for clients who do not respond to side spoon feeding, slight downward pressure on the front 1/3 of the tongue may facilitate tongue retraction and tongue bowl shape. However, if this technique facilitates tongue protrusion, discontinue immediately. This is a technique that is mainly useful for adults who have suffered a neurological infarction and need dysphagia therapy. It is most often contraindicated in pediatric patients because of the risk of provoking a tongue thrust.

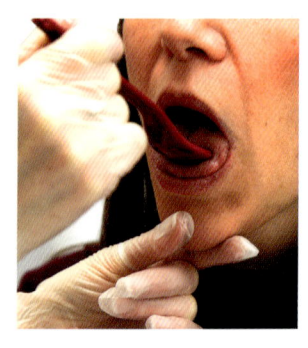

A Sensory Motor Approach to Feeding

PLACEMENT

5. Syringe Feeding - If significant tongue protrusion persists with therapeutic feeding techniques, syringe feeding may be used. Present 1-2 cc of a favorite puree in the buccal cavity at approximately the first molar (or where it would insert). Jaw support can be provided with your non dominant hand if necessary. Alternate sides and repeat for 4-5 repetitions on each side.

SUPPORT

1. If the client needs head, jaw, cheek, and lip support, consider the "v" support described at the beginning of this chapter.

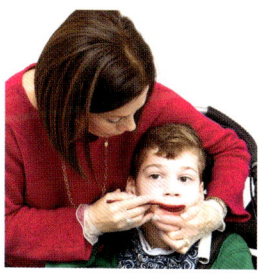

2. If your client only needs jaw/lower lip support, the feeder can be in front of the client, seated so that the feeder is below his/her gaze, or even within his/her gaze. (Note: If the feeder is above the client, the eater will need to look up, and vision drives movement. As gaze is directed upward, he/she will move the head into extension.) In this position, use the "c" support as mentioned at the start of this chapter.

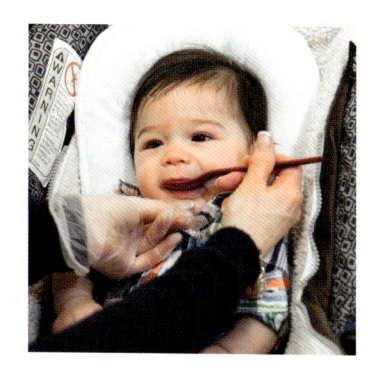

Chapter 9: Therapeutic Feeding

150

Cubes

Small cubes of solid foods are typically introduced between 7 and 9 months of age. Typically developing babies may initially suck, then use a non-dissociated munch-chew, followed by the acquisition of lateral tongue movement, to facilitate oral transport to the molar ridge for mastication. Then, tongue lateralization across midline develops, and finally, a rotary chew pattern emerges.

Prerequisite Skills: The typically developing baby has a rhythmic up/down bite with solid foods. This is followed by active transfer of food from the side of the mouth to the center or from the center to the side. Mobility through the tongue tip and lateral border of the tongue supports transfer of the food from the front of the mouth to the chewing surface. Then, tongue lateralization across midline and diagonal rotary jaw movement develops over time.

Clinical Suggestions

- If your client is an independent eater, take turns during meal or snack time, so that you are maintaining independence while facilitating improved sensory-motor skills. You may need to start therapeutic feeding programs slowly.
- If the techniques make mealtime longer, begin with 4-5 repetitions of therapeutic feeding at each meal.
- Encourage families to proceed with nutritive feeding. As a client accommodates, slowly increase the repetitions at each meal by one trial on each side at a time.
- While everyone has a stronger or dominant jaw side, if the client ignores one side completely, you may need to double the repetitions on the weaker side.
- For all positions, the feeder should be eye level or below the child to ensure the maintenance of appropriate head/neck posture.

POSITION	A client should be placed in a well-supported seated position with hips at a 90-degree angle, knees at a 90-degree angle, feet grounded, head in alignment, hands at midline. Clients with high tone may benefit from having support under their knees. Any of the high chairs, booster seats, therapeutic feeding chairs, or adaptive wheelchairs discussed in the spoon feeding section may be appropriate.
FOODS	For most toddlers, the first solid foods are easy to masticate, solids such as Gerber® Puffs, Mum Mums®, Cheerios® etc. For toddlers with allergies or children with intolerances, cubes of easy to masticate vegetables (sweet potato, squash) or fruits (banana, cooked apple) may be used. For more information, see cubed solids in the *Oral Sensory-Motor Cookbook* or in the Gluten Free Casein Free (GFCF) supplement found in the Appendix section of this text.
UTENSILS	A gloved hand or a cocktail-style fork. Coffee stirrers and plastic toothpicks are alternative utensils for clients who do not have seizures or a tonic bite.

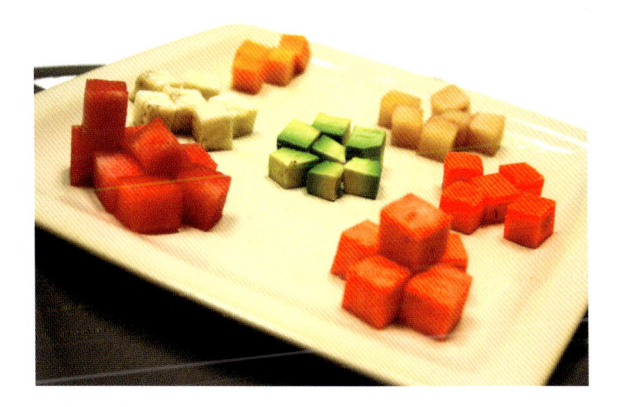

PLACEMENT

1. Food should be placed on the lateral molar ridge about where the first molar is (or will insert see "B"). With infants (or children who don't automatically begin to chew) place the cube on the molar ridge (B) and provide slight downward pressure to facilitate a munch-chew. When the child starts to munch remove your finger/fork. If the food falls in the middle of the tongue (and your client does not have teeth), use a gloved hand to help sweep it back to the molar ridge (B).

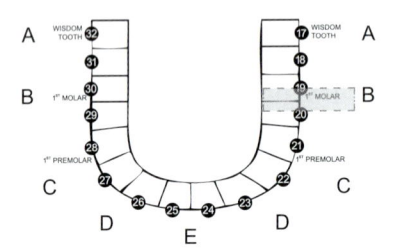

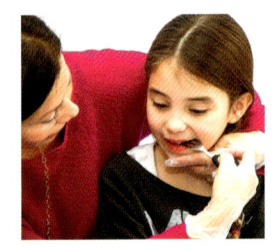

2. With many children or adults you can use a European fork technique. Spear a cube of food on a cocktail fork and present it European style (upside down) on the first molar (Position B). Use jaw support with your non dominant hand, if needed. Alternate sides. Everyone has a dominant side of the mouth for chewing; however, if your client ignores one side of the mouth, or has noticeable weakness on one side (e.g., Bell's Palsy), it is recommended to do two reps on the weaker side and one repetition on the stronger side.

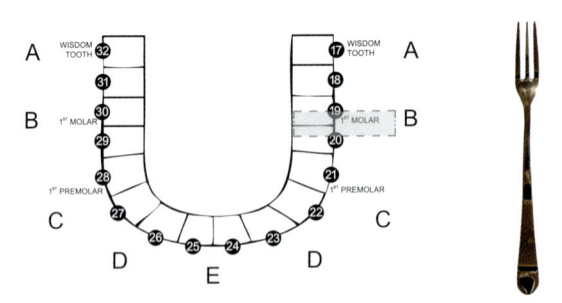

Note: If you are working with children who have teeth and are just learning to eat solids, the feeder needs to control the bolus. In this case start with a stick-shaped bolus using the chewing hierarchy. Return to cube feeding once your client has a repetitive lateral chew.

A Sensory Motor Approach to Feeding

SUPPORT — Hopefully you have worked on the motor plan for chewing in your pre-feeding program, and the client will not need jaw and lip support. However, if necessary, place a finger under the mandible and a finger under the lower lip to provide stability for chewing (see "V" support).

Strips

Typically developing children are offered cookies, teething biscuits, etc., around 7-9 months of age. Typically developing babies may initially suck, then use a non-dissociated munch chew, followed by the acquisition of lateral tongue movement, to facilitate oral transport to the molar ridge for mastication. Then, tongue lateralization across midline develops, and finally, a rotary chew pattern emerges.

Prerequisite Skills: The typically developing baby has a rhythmic up/down bite with solid foods. This is followed by active transfer of food from the side of the mouth to the center or from the center to the side. Mobility through the tongue tip and lateral border of the tongue supports transfer of the food from the front of the mouth to the chewing surface. Then tongue lateralization across midline and diagonal rotary jaw movement develops over time.

Clinical Suggestions

- If your client is an independent eater, take turns during meal or snack time so that you are maintaining independence while facilitating improved sensory-motor skills. You may need to start therapeutic feeding programs slowly.
- If the techniques make mealtime longer, begin with 4-5 repetitions of therapeutic feeding at each meal.
- Encourage families to proceed with nutritive feeding. As a client accommodates, slowly increase the repetitions at each meal by one trial on each side at a time.
- While everyone has a stronger or dominant jaw side, if the client ignores one side completely, you may need to double the repetitions on the weaker side.
- For all positions, the feeder should be eye level or below the child to ensure the maintenance of appropriate head/neck posture.

POSITION	A client should be placed in a well-supported seated position with the hips at a 90-degree angle, knees at a 90-degree angle, feet grounded, head in alignment, hands at midline. Clients with high tone may benefit from having support under their knees. Any of the highchairs, booster seats, therapeutic feeding chairs, or adaptive wheelchairs discussed in the spoon feeding section may be appropriate.
FOODS	Choose a stick-shaped bolus as described in Appendix B of the Oral-Sensory-motor Cookbook. Examples are: Veggie Sticks, Cheeto®, Jicama, thin apple strips, thin yucca fries, sweet potato fries, waffle, French toast, or a French fry. For children with dietary considerations, refer to Appendix A.
UTENSILS	Gloved hand
PLACEMENT	The Chewing Hierarchy

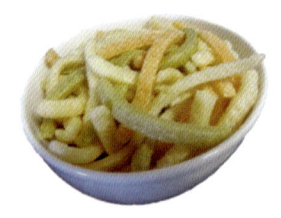

The Chewing Hierarchy was designed to sequence the oral sensory-motor skills for eating solid foods. It is important to be working on developing the oral sensory-motor skills in pre-feeding prior to introducing foods. For example, for a child who has not developed a munch chew, he/she is on pre-feeding Chewing Hierarchy Level 1 with an appropriate tool, and solids have not yet been introduced. Once the child has mastered pre-feeding Chewing Hierarchy Level 1, and has moved to Chewing Hierarchy Level 2 on the appropriate tool, then easy to masticate solids can be started at Chewing Hierarchy Level 1 for feeding. The same Chewing Hierarchy is used for both pre-feeding (non-edibles) and feeding. The following represents the relationship of the Chewing Hierarchy with non-edibles and edibles:

Pre-Feeding Hierarchy (non-edibles)	Feeding Hierarchy (edibles)
Chewing Hierarchy Level 1 with Red/Yellow Chewy Tubes®, Z-Vibe® with an appropriate tip	Solids have not been introduced
Chewing Hierarchy Level 2 with Red/Yellow Chewy Tubes®, Z-Vibe® with an appropriate tip	Strips Chewing Hierarchy Level 1
Chewing Hierarchy Level 3 with Yellow Chewy Tubes®	Strips Chewing Hierarchy Level 2
Chewing Hierarchy Level 4 with Red/Yellow Chewy Tubes®, Z-Vibe® with an appropriate tip	Strips Chewing Hierarchy Level 3
	Strips Chewing Hierarchy Level 4

The selection of the tool reflects the child's oral sensory-motor system. If the child has no teeth, a toothette dipped in ice or a favorite puree/juice may be used. If a child is under-responsive to input and over a year of age, a vibration tool, such as a Z-Vibe® with a blue tip, may be used. If a child benefits from deep pressure, a Chewy Tube® may be selected. For a child with a high fixed jaw posture, start with the yellow Chewy Tube®. If the child is in a low, poorly graded jaw posture, the red Chewy Tube® may be a better choice. The red Chewy Tube® is softer and easier to compress, and the yellow Chewy Tube® is slightly firmer. Take this into consideration if your client has reduced jaw strength. The goal is that a child can do Chewing Hierarchy Level 1 for 4-5 repetition x 2 sets, with both yellow and red Chewy Tubes®.

EXERCISE	TARGET GROUPS	GOALS	TOOLS
Feeding Chewing Hierarchy 1	4-6 months and up	Symmetrical Chew Tongue Retraction Lateral Chew	Stick shaped bolus (see pages 199 and 205)

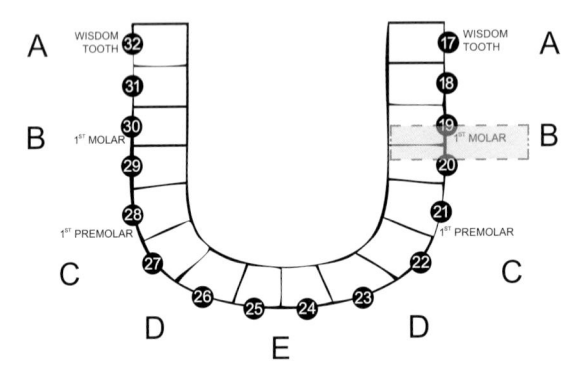

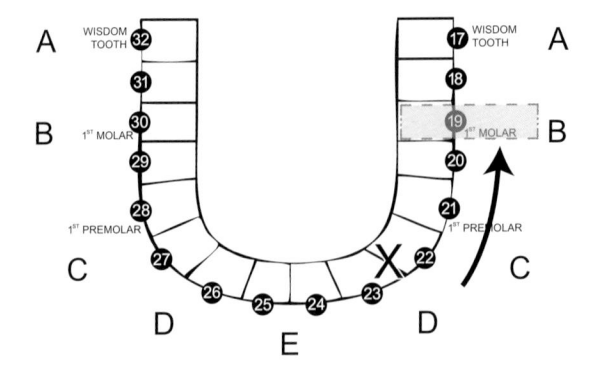

Present the stick shaped bolus to the lateral molar ridge where the first molar will insert (B). Provide firm pressure into the tool to stimulate a munch chew. If necessary, support the jaw with your non dominant hand. Work toward 4-5 repetitive bites on one side and then the other. Repeat this cycle 2x.

EXERCISE	TARGET GROUPS	GOALS	TOOLS
Feeding Chewing Hierarchy 2	7-9 months and up	Tongue Tip Pointing Lateral Chew (diagonal)	Stick shaped bolus (see pages 199 and 205)

A Sensory Motor Approach to Feeding

Present the stick shaped bolus to the lateral incisor (or where it would insert) at "D." Facilitate a bite on the lateral incisor and immediately move the bolus to the location of the first molar (B) and facilitate a second bite. Repeat 4-5x on one side and then the other. The therapist should look for tongue lateralization from the lateral incisor (D) to the first molar (B).

EXERCISE	TARGET GROUPS	GOALS	TOOLS
Feeding Chewing Hierarchy 3	10-12 months and up	Crossing the midline Reduce extraneous head movement secondary to unresolved rooting	Stick shaped bolus (see pages 199 and 205)

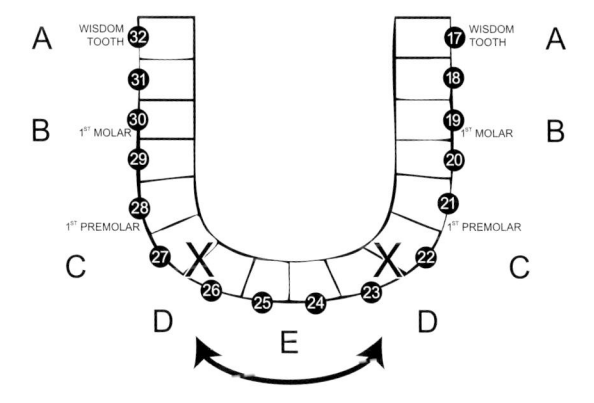

Present one stick shaped bolus on the client's lateral incisor (D) and facilitate a bite. Immediately present the second stick shaped bolus on the opposite lateral incisor and facilitate a bite (D). Work left to right and right to left 4-5 repetitions x 2 sets. The use of two stick shaped boluses reduces rooting and extraneous head movements, and encourages jaw stability and a dissociated bite.

EXERCISE	TARGET GROUPS	GOALS	TOOLS
Feeding Chewing Hierarchy 4	13-15 months and up	Motor plan for a rotary chew	Stick shaped bolus (see pages 199 and 205)

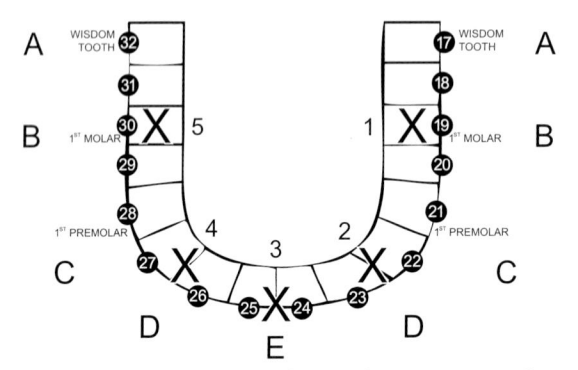

Present the food of choice on the client's first molar (B1). Provide stability with your non dominant hand as needed. Encourage the client to do 5 small graded bites: first molar (B1), lateral incisor (D2), front central incisor (E3), lateral incisor (D4), and first molar (B5) on the opposite side. 4-5x right to left, 4-5x left to right for 2 sets. Note that everyone has a stronger side; however, if your client has significant weakness on one side you may work 2x on the weaker side as opposed to 1x on the stronger side.

SUPPORT

Jaw support can be imposed, if necessary, using the "v" support position.

Cup

Open-cup drinking can be introduced therapeutically as early as 5-6 months of age with supports. Open-cup drinking is not nutritive at this point; it is meant to develop oral sensory-motor skills. The goal is to help a baby develop the oral sensory-motor skills to eliminate bottle feeding between a year and 15 months of age. Sippy cups should only be used if there are no other options for hydrating a client (Eig, 2002). A sippy cup is stabilized with the tongue (much like a bottle nipple), and a suckle is used to draw liquid. Reducing tongue protrusion is the goal of transitioning a child to a cup.

Prerequisite Skills: Jaw stability and grading, lip closure, cheek contraction, and tongue retraction

Clinical Suggestions
- If your client is an independent eater, take turns during meal or snack time so that you are maintaining independence while facilitating improved sensory-motor skills. You may need to start therapeutic feeding programs slowly.
- If the techniques make mealtime longer, begin with 4-5 repetitions of therapeutic feeding at each meal.
- Encourage families to proceed with nutritive feeding. As a client accommodates, slowly increase the repetitions at each meal by one trial on each side at a time.
- For all positions, the feeder should be eye level or below the child to ensure the maintenance of appropriate head/neck posture.

POSITION

If you are starting open-cup drinking with an infant, you may need to provide support by holding the infant on your lap to stabilize the body and use the "V" support to provide head, jaw, and lower lip supports. Children and adults may be in a well supported seated position as described in spoon feeding. It is important to maintain the head in neutral flexion for cup drinking.

FOODS

1. For infants, nectar consistency is recommended. Traditionally rice cereal was used to thicken formula; however for a variety of reasons this is now contraindicated (Knox, 2008). The amylase in breast milk breaks down the rice and increases caloric content, and shifting the balance of nutrients. It decreases motility, increases constipation, and may decrease hydration. In addition, the safety of commercial thickeners

FOODS

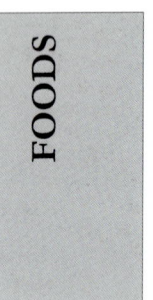

has been questioned, especially in premature infants. Whenever possible, change the viscosity of the liquid naturally, i.e., by increasing the powder to water ratio in formula, or by thinning out a puree.

2. For toddlers, Stage 1 consistency baby fruits or vegetables can be thinned to nectar consistency with spring water. Fruit smoothies are another option.

UTENSILS

1. The cut-out cup facilitates lip closure and tongue retraction while allowing the client to maintain the head in neutral flexion.

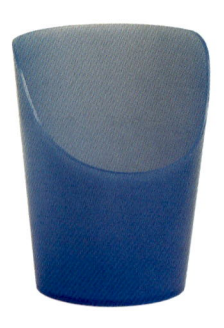

2. As children become more independent, consider a recessed lid cup or an infa trainer cup. These utensils will allow the child to maintain the head in neutral flexion.

RECESSED LID CUP   INFA TRAINER CUP

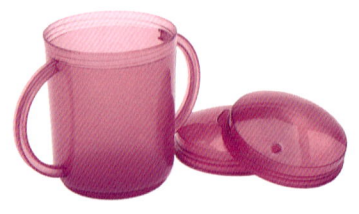

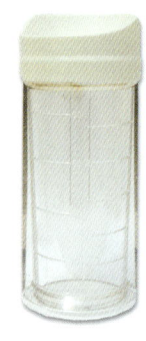

A Sensory Motor Approach to Feeding

PLACEMENT

The cup should be on the client's lower lip, just contacting the corners of the lips. The shape of the cup should allow the client to draw liquid without requiring head/neck extension. When cup drinking is initially introduced, work on single repetitive sips.

1. Place the cup rim to the client's lower lip.

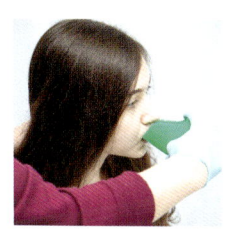

2. Roll the cup upward while maintaining labial contact, while the client takes one sip.

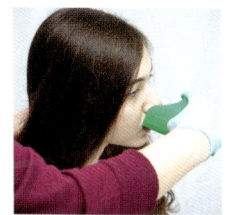

3. Roll the cup back to the neutral position while maintaining labial contact.

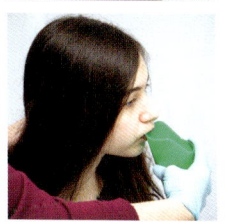

Repeat this cycle, and slowly increase the amount of sips until the client can draw multiple, repetitive sips.

SUPPORT

"V" or "C" supports

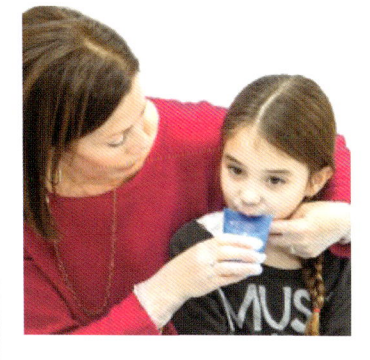

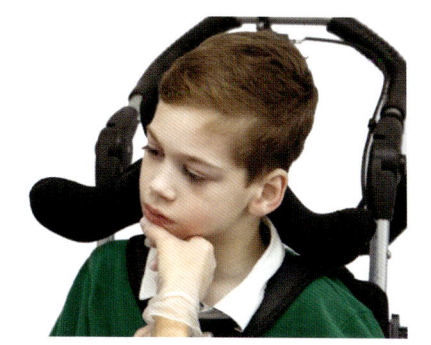

Chapter 9: Therapeutic Feeding

162

Straw

Do not introduce the cup and straw simultaneously. Usually the cup is first. If a strong lingual protrusion cannot be addressed with supports during cup drinking, try therapeutic straw drinking first. Straw drinking can be introduced as early as six to seven months (Bahr, 2010) but is usually introduced at about 10 months of age.

Prerequisite Skills: Jaw stability and grading for a high jaw position, lip rounding with tongue retraction, and cheek contraction.

Clinical Suggestions

- If your client is an independent eater, take turns during meal or snack time so that you are maintaining independence while facilitating improved sensory-motor skills. You may need to start therapeutic feeding programs slowly.
- If the techniques make mealtime longer, begin with 4-5 repetitions of therapeutic feeding at each meal.
- Encourage families to proceed with nutritive feeding. As a client accommodates, slowly increase the repetitions at each meal by one trial on each side at a time.
- For all positions, the feeder should be eye level or below the child to ensure the maintenance of appropriate head/neck posture.

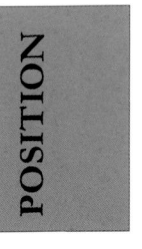

POSITION

A well supported seated position
(see spoon, cube, strip, or cup)

FOODS

1. Water or slightly thickened nectar consistency liquid. For example, thin out a Stage 1 fruit with bottled water.

2. Carbonated beverages can provide sensory feedback.

FOODS

3. Cold drinks can help contract the muscles.

4. Pungent flavors such as lemonade, cranberry juice, or tamarind nectar also provide increased sensory information for older clients.

UTENSILS

1. **Honey Bear Straw Cup** (or for an older child or adult use a squeeze bottle fitted with oxygen tubing): The Honey Bear allows the therapist to provide jaw and lip cues while gently squeezing small amounts of liquid into the oral cavity. Jaw and cheek support may initially be needed to teach straw drinking. The "C" support is helpful while using this tool. The Honey Bear Straw Cup comes with complete directions from TalkTools®.

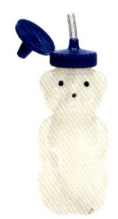

2. **Sip-Tip Cup:** This tool is designed for individuals with weakened intraoral suctioning.

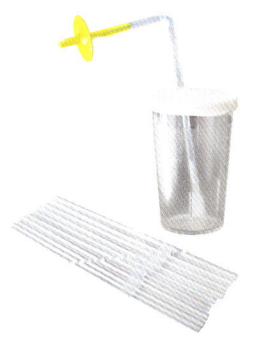

3. Once the child is straw drinking, **The TalkTools® Straw Hierarchy** is recommended for targeting lip rounding, lip protrusion, tongue retraction, and jaw-lip-tongue dissociation (Rosenfeld-Johnson, 2006).

Chapter 9: Therapeutic Feeding

PLACEMENT

1. Place the tubing on the client's lower lip. If he/she can maintain tongue retraction with jaw support then begin in this manner. Provide a small graded sip by squeezing the bottle with your non dominant hand and assist your client in maintaining jaw stability so they can achieve tongue retraction and lip closure for a swallow. Work towards 5-6 single repetitive sips. Do not remove the straw.

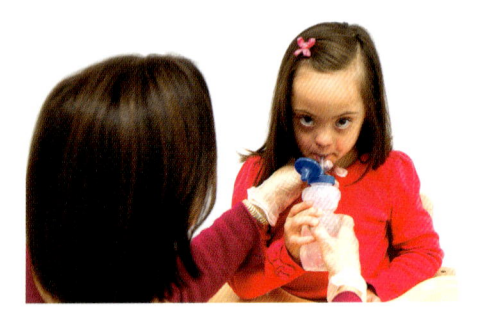

2. If a strong lingual protrusion persists, place the tubing in the buccal cavity, at approximately position C.

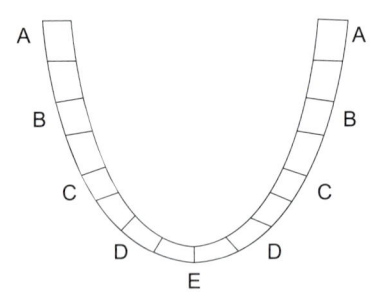

Provide jaw/lip support and give a small, graded sip. Alternate sides and repeat. Once your client can maintain lip closure to swallow, move from side to side, then middle, and eventually to just the middle. Start with single sips and work up to repetitive sips as your client can manage this process.

SUPPORT

1. "V" or "C" supports.

2. Note that when introducing straw drinking with infants, you will need to provide support.

CONCLUSION:

The goal of a therapeutic feeding program is to develop the oral sensory-motor skills for safe, effective, nutritive feeding. This chapter has focused on therapeutic feeding hierarchy, including: position, food choices/sensory-motor diet shaping, food placement, utensils, and supports that are all important in developing a program plan. The prerequisite skills for breast, bottle, cube, strip, cup, and straw drinking have been defined. The pre-feeding program is desirably one step ahead of the therapeutic feeding program to develop the oral sensory-motor skills needed to support therapeutic feeding. Now that we have assessed a client and established a foundation of both pre-feeding and feeding tasks, we are ready to write a report, which will be outlined in Chapter 10.

CHAPTER 10:
PROGRAM PLANNING AND CASE STUDIES

LEADING GOALS/POINTS

Learning to write a report

Generating an evaluation and Program Plan

Reviewing sample case studies

Now that the assessment has been completed, you are ready to write a report and create a treatment plan (Chapters 6-9).

First, you will complete this checklist to ensure that you have gathered all the necessary information:

- Case history
- Medical information
- Previous reports
- 5-day baseline diet
- Structural assessment
- Posture and alignment assessment
- Positioning and seating assessment
- Pre-feeding skills assessment
- Feeding skills assessment

Next, you will write a report. We will follow three children from assessment to program planning.

1. Sean, a 3.11-year-old male with a diagnosis of bilateral open-lip schizencephaly (a type of cleft in the brain caused by cerebral cortical malformations) and right hemiparesis (right-sided weakness due to an injury to the left brain).

2. Joe, a 3-year-old male with a diagnosis of Autism Spectrum Disorder.

3. John, a 3.2-year-old male with a diagnosis of Down Syndrome.

There will be six sections in each report: 1) Identifying data; 2) Background Information; 3) Testing Observations; 4) Summary and Recommendations; 5) Program Plan; and 6) Goals and Objectives.

Sample Report Writing

FOR FULL REPORTS, SEE APPENDIX E

1) Identifying Data

The first part of the report is a heading that lists important client information.

Case #1

Name: Sean Martin	DOB: 1/1/08
Address: 32 Main Street City, State Zip	Chronological Age: 3.11
Phone: 201.545.1211	Parents Names: Sean and Maria Martin
Primary Physician: Dr. Kim	Referring Physician: Dr. Kim
Diagnosis: bilateral open-lip schizencephaly and right hemiparesis	Procedure Code: 92610

Case #2

Name: Joe Perez	DOB: 3/21/09
Address: 32 Main Street City, State Zip	Chronological Age: 3 years
Phone: 201.545.1211	Parents Names: Juan and Mary Perez
Primary Physician: Dr. Broderick	Referring Physician: n/a school based referral
Diagnosis: Autism Spectrum Disorder	Procedure Code: 92610

Case # 3

Name: John Jones	DOB: 2/1/09
Address: 32 Main Street City, State Zip	Chronological Age: 3.2
Phone: 201.545.1200	Parents Names: Jeff and Kelly Jones
Primary Physician: Dr. Patel	Referring Physician: Dr. Patel
Diagnosis: Down syndrome	Procedure Code: 92610

2) Background Information

The following are three examples of background information to be included in a report. In this section you will report all the information you gathered, including the birth, medical, developmental, educational, sensory, nutritional, and feeding information discussed in Chapters 2-5. This can be written in a narrative or bulleted format:

CASE #1: SEAN

Sean, a 3.11 year old boy with a diagnosis of bilateral open lip schizencephaly/right hemiparesis was seen for an oral motor/feeding evaluation. Sean was accompanied by his mother and grandparents, who served as informants. Sean was referred for this evaluation by Dr. Kim, secondary to concerns about safe, nutritive feeding.

Sean is the product of a full-term pregnancy and uncomplicated delivery. Neonatal course was reportedly uneventful. Early motor development was a concern and, at 10 months of age, Sean was diagnosed with bilateral open-lip schizencephaly and right hemiparesis. Medical history is significant for constipation. Sean has had Botox treatments on his right arm and leg, which have yielded positive results with mobility. More recently, he had Botox treatments on his salivary glands to decrease drooling. However, there have not been notable changes in saliva control.

Sean was successfully bottle-fed and transitioned to purees without incident. He reportedly has always been a messy eater and loses food on the right side of his mouth. Sean's solid foods are limited by his mother and grandparents secondary to safety concerns. Soft solids are cut into very small pieces, as Sean "does not really chew well." Raw vegetables, meat, crunchy snacks (chips), hard fruit, and bagels, are difficult for Sean. He drinks from an open cup and a straw. He is more successful with a toddler sippy cup. To date, he has not had a specific pre-feeding program. His family has been told to "rub a Z-Vibe® on his face and in his mouth" prior to feeding.

CASE #2: JOE

Family History: Joe resides in Fairlawn, NJ, with his father (age 39), a stockbroker and his mother (age 33), a homemaker. He is an only child. English and Spanish are spoken in the home. There is history of a speech delay on the maternal side of the family, and Mr. Perez has a history of a hearing loss. There is a history of cancer, on both the paternal and maternal sides of the family.

Birth History: Joe was born at 37 weeks gestation. Preeclampsia was diagnosed and required hospitalization. His mother's pregnancy was negative for smoking, drugs, and alcohol use. After a long labor, Joe was born via C-section, secondary to fetal distress. His birth weight was 8 lbs 4 ounces, and he had an Apgar Score of 8. His blood sugar was low at birth (54).

Medical History: Joe has not been hospitalized since birth. He has a history of sinus infections and croup. He has no known allergies. He sees a physician regularly and has a developmental pediatrician, who diagnosed him with "Moderate Autism." His hearing was tested and by parent report, was within normal limits.

Developmental History: Joe's gross motor skills were reportedly normal.

He also babbled and spoke his first words on time, seven months and one year respectively. He is starting to form sentences recently. His mother reported that he can read multiple words, learned his alphabet by 21 months, can count up to 40, and has a good memory.

Oral and Feeding History: Joe was described as "a very picky eater." His parents expressed concern with his diet. To supplement Joe, he is given Pediasure in a bottle at night. Mrs. Perez stated that Joe drinks this throughout the nighttime hours and is offered bottles in his crib. He never sucked his thumb or liked a pacifier. He sometimes tenses his jaw/grinds his teeth. He exhibits an open-mouth posture at times.

Sensory History: Sensory-based issues were not reported by Joe's parents, yet they were noted at school, especially in the oral sensory-motor domain. He also reportedly covers his ears during school announcements, and during gym and music.

Social History: He was described by his parents as "happy, friendly, and playful." He reportedly takes some time to interact in social settings. He enjoys puzzles, the iPad, trucks, and sand.

CASE #3: JOHN

John is a 3.2-year-old boy with a diagnosis of Down Syndrome. He was seen for an oral sensory-motor/feeding evaluation. John was accompanied by his parents, who served as informants.

John is the product of a full-term pregnancy. His complicated medical history includes cardiac failure at three weeks of age. John had open heart surgery (patent ductus arteriosis/PDA repair) at three months of age. John has a history of reflux and chronic constipation. He also has a history of upper respiratory infections and bronchiolitis. At nine months of age, he had a gastrointestinal tube placed. John also has a diagnosis of hypothyroidism. John wears glasses to correct nearsightedness and

has a hearing aid to address bilateral conductive loss.
John's feeding history was reported as follows:

- At birth John breast fed well.

- Following cardiac failure, he fatigued easily and had to be supplemented with syringe feeding.

- Nasogastric (NG) feeds were initiated with John following cardiac admission.

- Reflux worsened with nasogastric (NG) tube feeds.

- Breast feeding was reintroduced at nine months of age, post surgery. John had a weak suck, and his ability to latch had deteriorated. Cup feeding and spoon feeding were initiated, but feeding took up to an hour, and John failed to gain adequate weight.

- Enteral feeds were reintroduced. In May of 2009, a percutaneous endoscopic gastrostomy (PEG) tube was inserted.

- John participated in a three-week PEG tube weaning program at 30 months of age. He transitioned to high calorie Fortini drinks and pureed textures.

- Since that time, John has participated in feeding therapy, and John's mother has been instructed to increase the texture of his food. John reportedly swallows textured foods without chewing. He gags/vomits when food becomes "stuck" on his tongue.

3) Testing Observations

The testing observation section or "discussion," as it is often labeled, is the bulk of the report. This includes both subjective and objective observations and the results of pre-feeding and therapeutic feeding interventions utilized to gather information (Chapters 7 and 9). In most cases, it is beneficial to film/record this section of the evaluation, so parents have examples of the therapeutic strategies used during the assessment. This will help the parents, or treating therapist, understand the recommendations and program plan.

CASE #1: SEAN

Sean's evaluation and summary were recorded on video for his family and team. The following is an overview of the clinical observations:

- Sean presented with posture and muscle tone issues which impacted feeding and speech. He had shortened pectoralis muscles, decreased rib cage mobility, flared ribs, and decreased abdominal/oblique support for controlled respiration. Respiration was shallow and did not support more than one or two words at a time. Tone in the oral musculature was reduced, but movement patterns in the lips and tongue reflect extensor patterns.

- Sean had a high palatal vault.

- Sean's jaw symmetry, strength, and stability were notably compromised. Jaw sliding was observed at rest. A non-dissociated, poorly graded munch chew (with food forward in the oral cavity) was observed with all textures. Wide jaw excursions were noted with chewing, sucking on a sippy cup nipple, and sound production. Sean does not have adequate strength to masticate a solid bolus, and he often swallowed food that was not adequately broken down/chewed. There was no evidence of emerging jaw/lip/tongue dissociation or grading for feeding or sound production.

- The buccal musculature was poorly defined, and Sean did not use his cheeks to support sucking, chewing, swallowing, stabilizing a solid bolus, or sound production.

- The labial musculature was retracted at rest and during support function. Sean did not have functional bilateral approximation for spoon feeding. He bit the spoon and cleared the bolus with a non-dissociated trunk, shoulder, neck, jaw movement. He did not approximate lip closure during chewing. Labial seal on a straw or cup was poor (particularly on the right side), and Sean compensated by using his tongue.

- The lingual musculature was bulgy and poorly defined. Sean did not use the lateral borders of his tongue or tongue tip functionally. Sean's primary lingual movement continued to be a suckle (protrusion/retraction). He used this pattern along with tongue dumping to move a solid bolus. Food is transported to the canine (not the first molar) for mastication. Food fell onto the lingual surface and was suckled at midline. The bolus was handled in the front third of the mouth and was often spread across the tongue.

- With regard to sensory processing, Sean clearly had reduced awareness both inside and outside of the mouth. He was a copious drooler and is seemingly unaware of saliva running down his chin. He stuffed his mouth, and sought salty high-taste foods. Sean frequently did not clear a solid bolus and residual food pooled on the lateral borders of the tongue and within his palate. Sean also "stopped chewing" with residual food in his mouth and appeared to be unaware of food held intra-orally.

- Sean took a long time to break down food and often swallowed a poorly masticated bolus. This presented a significant choking risk.

CASE #2: JOE

Joe had limited eye contact. He preferred to sit at a work table rather than explore the room. During snack time in the classroom, he was anxious. He often pushed his chair away from the table and recited songs and the ABCs. He became anxious at lunch time and started to cry, which does not happen during the day. Joe did not like to touch the foods presented, and preferred to be fed.

Joe was seen across several therapy sessions starting in mid-October and concluding 11/16/11. Assessment was challenging because he had intermittent illness and missed many days at school. Upon returning to school, he refused to eat. His oral sensory-motor issues made intraoral assessment quite difficult. After several sessions the following was revealed:

1. Joe appeared to have anxiety when presented with food, even foods he preferred.

2. Structural assessment revealed: fatty sucking pads, decreased buccal tone, upper lip pulling upward toward the nasal philtrum, open mouth posture, decreased lingual muscle tone, an overbite, weak jaw strength, indentia (i.e. spacing between the top central incisors), and poor oral resting posture.

3. Feeding skill assessment revealed: tongue thrusting, poor jaw-lip-tongue dissociation and grading, slow eating speed, constant raking of food (top teeth to bottom lip), and decreased sensory awareness.

4. Oral Placement skills were marked by: decreased oral sensory awareness, increased tactile defensiveness, poor phonatory control, poor jaw stability, weak jaw-lip-tongue dissociation, and poor speech intelligibility beyond the word level.

5. Joe had a self-limited diet as established by his 5-day profile:

	10/24/11	10/25/11	10/26/11	10/27/11	10/28/11
BREAKFAST	1/4 cup rice cereal and OJ	3 bites of apple-flavored cereal bar, waffle	small amount of rice cereal and OJ	white bread, rice cereal and OJ	apple-flavored cereal, oatmeal cookie
SNACK	0	0	0	0	0
LUNCH	1 piece chicken patty, 1 spoon mac and cheese and water	2-3 ounces mac and cheese, 2 oatmeal cookies and OJ	2-3 ounces mac and cheese and water	half portion mac and cheese	OJ
DINNER	1 portion (10) of homemade french fries, refused all other options and OJ	3 chicken nuggets, 1/2 portion of fries and OJ	5 chicken nuggets, fries, OJ, rice and mac and cheese	refused dinner drank 8 ounces of Pediasure®	refuses dinner and liquids
SNACK	0	1 cookie	0	0	0

6. Home Base diet revealed that Joe eats a variety of textures, but prefers bland and sweet foods. Visual presentation also seems important as he wants his food to always look the same and familiar. He breaks foods apart and does not seem to "like" his foods, or enjoy meals.

CASE #3: JOHN

This evaluation was requested to assess John's oral sensory-motor skill development to support safe, nutritive feeding with solid foods. John's evaluation and summary were recorded on video by his father. The following is an overview of the clinical observations:

- John presented with notably decreased postural stability. He is not yet walking. In a seated position he relied on a wide base of support. He fixed secondary to reduced stability (using one hand to stabilize as he used the other hand, fixing with his shoulders in a high posture as he reached, teeth grinding to stabilize his jaw, etc.). John's head was often in extension. He had shortened pectoral muscles, abducted scapulas, and flared ribs. The majority of his movements persisted in the sagittal plane.

A comprehensive evaluation with an NDT certified physical therapist was strongly recommended.

- Muscle tone was decreased peri and intra-orally. This was consistent with muscle tone throughout his body.

- John was in a habitual open-mouth posture with a retracted upper lip. Lip closure for spoon feeding was accomplished with jaw/lower lip movement. John did not have functional lip rounding during straw drinking or speech sound production.

- John's lingual musculature (i.e., tongue) sits low and forward. John often protruded his tongue past his front central incisors at rest and to support function. John did not use the lateral borders of his tongue or his tongue tip during feeding or speech. A protraction-retraction persisted as John's primary lingual movement. It should be noted that lingual alveolar sounds are produced with the tongue blade contacting his front central incisors.

- John's strength and stability in the buccal musculature were compromised. John did not use his cheeks to support sucking or swallowing. Mobility in the buccal musculature was not adequate to support chewing or to stabilize a solid bolus.

- John's jaw strength and stability were compromised. John did not have a functional non-nutritive or nutritive chew. He could bite and hold, but it was difficult to establish a repetitive "chew" pattern. The sensory-motor plan for repetitive chewing was facilitated with alternating chewy tubes (i.e., the clinician placed a Chewy Tube® on each molar, rotating right to left and left to right, in an effort to assess if John could alternate sides. He was not successful).

- John presented with oral sensory issues. He was reportedly defensive to input both outside and inside the mouth (i.e., massage, or tooth brushing). During our three sessions he demonstrated the ability to accommodate to oral sensory-motor input when it was paired with whole body input. It should be noted that sensory defensiveness may develop secondary to negative experiences.

- John used a repetitive reverse swallow pattern to handle purees and exaggerated tongue protrusion to handle liquids.

4) Summary

The report summary reviews the pertinent data and concludes a diagnosis and therapy recommendations.

CASE #1: SEAN

Sean presents with neuro-motor, muscle tone, and oral sensory-motor issues that clearly impact both feeding and speech. He has made great gains in gross and fine motor development. Significant challenges persist in both feeding and speech sound production.

The following program plan was developed to address the development of oral sensory-motor skills to support safe, effective, nutritive feeding.

I would be happy to work with Sean's family and team as this plan is implemented. I can best be reached via email at feedingslp@123.com. Sean's mother and grandmother will update me periodically via email. I would like to re-evaluate Sean in approximately four months to assess his progress and update his plan.

CASE #2: JOE

Joe has oral sensory-motor issues inhibiting his feeding skills, which has resulted in a self-limited diet. His poor eating habits are reinforced by allowing him bottles of Pediasure when he refuses solid foods. His delayed feeding skills are also the result of immature protraction/retraction action that he is using with the bottles. If Joe is going to improve his variety of temperature, texture, and taste, he will need to stop using the bottle and decrease liquid supplementation. We do not want to cause a situation where he is losing weight. Therefore, it is important that the pediatrician or a dietitian set caloric goals for Joe, so we can ensure he is eating enough calories every day to maintain his weight. He will require a pre-feeding plan to improve his oral sensory-motor skills as they relate to feeding.

CASE #3: JOHN

John is an engaging little boy who presents with significant delays in oral sensory-motor skill development to support safe, nutritive feeding with solid foods.

The following program plan was developed during a three-day feeding program. This plan should be implemented two to three times per day. I would be happy to consult with John's family and team as this plan is implemented. I can best be reached via email at feedingslp@123.com. John should be re-evaluated in approximately four months to assess his progress and update his plan.

5) Program Plan

The Program Plan is an outline and direction of pre-feeding and therapeutic feeding techniques to implement with the client. These activities are all included in Chapters 7 and 9 of this text.

CASE #1: SEAN

1. **Massage:** Start at the temporomandibular joint (TMJ) and provide firm, elongated massage to the corners of Sean's lips, alongside the nostrils into the insertion of the upper lip, and from under the nostrils into the upper lip. Do each set 4-5 times. Vary the sensory input and incorporate into daily living activities.

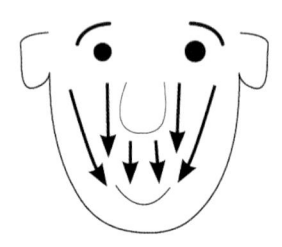

Sensory Suggestions:

- Bare hands – prior to meals, play
- Lotion – after bath
- Wet/dry washcloths – before/after meals, after bath
- Warm/cold washcloths – bath time
- Textured bean bags – play
- Vibration – play

This will increase sensory awareness and organization, encourage midline orientation, and facilitate increased cheek and upper lip mobility.

2. **Tap-n-Tone:** Provide firm, rhythmic tapping from the TMJ to the corners of the lips and on the surface of the lips to the beat of a favorite finger play activity or nursery rhyme.

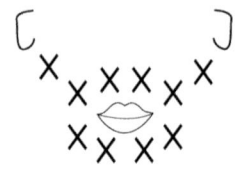

This will provide sensory input and tone to the buccal and labial musculature.

3. **Cheek Resistance with Slide:**

    A. Present the Z-Vibe® yellow preefer head in Sean's cheek and stretch out.

    B. Slide the tool to the corner of Sean's lips (like you are taking a lollipop out of his mouth) as you instruct him to kiss.

    C. As the tool comes to midline, instruct Sean to do a fish kiss. Do each "set" 5 times.

4. **Upper Lip Stretch:** You can do this exercise with a Z-Vibe® yellow preefer tip. Start under Sean's top lip and roll from the corner of the lip to midline. Stop. Repeat on the opposite side. Do each set 4-5 times.

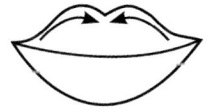

This will provide sensory input and increased upper lip mobility.

5. **Cheek Toning/Lip Rounding:** Present the rounded end of the Jiggler between his lips. Provide jaw/cheek support as needed to facilitate lip rounding. Model a [w] sound and encourage Sean to imitate. Repeat 10 times or as he will tolerate.

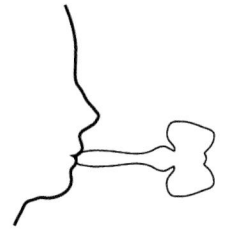

This will provide sensory input, facilitate increased tone in the cheeks, and encourage lip rounding.

6. **Bilateral Tongue Hugs:** You will need two Z-Vibes® small, square, green heads for this exercise. Present the Z-Vibes® bilaterally along the lateral borders of the tongue. Stroke firmly to the tongue tip. Repeat 5 times/2 sets.

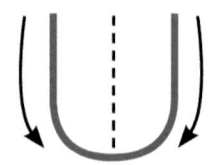

This will increase elongation through the lateral borders of the tongue and facilitate a tongue tip.

7. **Bilateral Chewy Tubes®:** (You will need two yellow and two red Chewy Tubes® for this exercise.)

   A. Present the yellow Chewy Tubes® bilaterally and perpendicular to the lateral molar ridges at the insertion of the back molars. Instruct Sean to do 10 slow, graded, repetitive bites. You may need to provide a visual model. Provide jaw support as demonstrated.

   B. Repeat with the red tubes.

This will increase jaw strength, jaw symmetry, tongue retraction, and graded movement.

Feeding:

1. **Spoon Feeding:** Use a vibrating spoon for purees. Turn the spoon sideways, contacting the corners of Sean's lips. Tilt the spoon slightly if you observe him biting the spoon.

This will encourage lip closure and tongue retraction.

A Sensory Motor Approach to Feeding

2. **Fork Feeding:** Use a cocktail-type/narrow fork for this exercise. Cut food into "Cheerio-sized" pieces and spear on the fork. Present the fork upside down and perpendicular to the lateral molar ridge. Alternate the side you present the fork on.

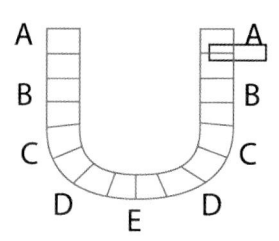

This will increase jaw grading, tongue retraction, and a lateral chew.

3. **Chewing Hierarchy:** Follow the directions on the protocol for Chewing Hierarchy Level #1 using a stick-shaped bolus. Alternate sides and repeat.

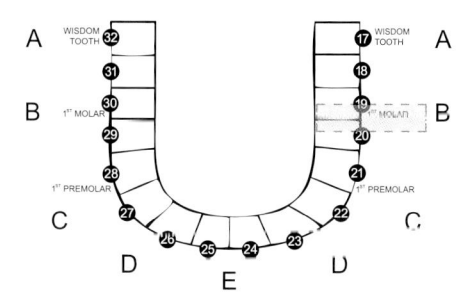

This will encourage a lateral chew, jaw grading, and tongue retraction.

4. **Straw Drinking:** Sean should be drinking from TalkTools® straw #1, cut to 1 inch above the animal head/lip block. Over the next several weeks soak the top of the straw in hot water and trim above the animal head/lip block. Eventually there should only be ¼ inch of straw above the animal head/lip block. Encourage him to do single sips.

This will increase lip rounding and tongue retraction.

Re-evaluation: Four months.

CASE #2: JOE

EXERCISE	TARGET GROUP	PHOTO	GOALS	TOOLS
Facial Massage	Any age Hyertonia Hypotonia		Sensory awareness Midline orientation Desensitizing for intra-oral stimulation Cheek mobility Lip mobility	Sensory bean bags Washcloth
Tapping	Any age Low tone only		Lip rounding Midline orientation Toning	Gloved finger
Myofascial Stretch and hold	Any age Hypotonia Upper lip insufficiency		Release for neuromuscular re-education Prerequisite for upper lip mobility	Gloved hand
Jiggler Roll	Any age 1+ Hypertonia Hypotonia		Upper lip mobility	Jiggler
Mouse Ears	Any age 1+ Hypertonia Hypotonia		Upper lip mobility Lip closure	Therapeutic Mouse Spoon Tip for the Z-Vibe®

CASE #2: JOE

EXERCISE	TARGET GROUP	PHOTO	GOALS	TOOLS
Corner to Midline Upper Lip Stretch	Any age Hypotonia Fixed upper lip		Upper lip mobility and strength	Trimmed toothette (non-flavored) Gloved finger Yellow Z-Vibe® tip Infadent
Vibrating Kisses	Any age 1+ Hypotonia		Cheek toning Lip rounding	Jiggler Electric toothbrush with a small round head
Cheek Stretch	Any age Requires active movement Hypotonia Hypertonia		Cheek mobility Lip strength Lip mobility Lip rounding For feeding and speech	Infadent Yellow Z-Vibe® tip Trimmed toothette (non-flavored)
Cheek Resistance	Any age Requires active movement Hypotonia Hypertonia		Cheek mobility Lip strength Lip mobility Lip rounding For feeding and speech	Infadent Yellow Z-Vibe® tip Trimmed toothette (non-flavored)
Cheek Toning Lip Rounding	Any age Requires active movement Hypotonia Hypertonia		Cheek toning Lip rounding For feeding and speech	Jiggler

CASE #2: JOE

EXERCISE	TARGET GROUP	PHOTO	GOALS	TOOLS
Fish Lip Pops	Any age Requires active movement		Cheek mobility Lip strength Lip mobility Lip rounding	Infadent Yellow Z-Vibe® tip
Maintaining Tongue Lateralization	Infant +		Provoke and maintain tongue lateralization	Z-Vibe® preefer tip
Lateral Tongue Massage	Any age 1+		Elongation of the tongue Tongue lateralization	Trimmed Toothette Z-Vibe® with fine tip (note: if there is jaw instability use Talk Tools® Bite Block level 6 or 7 to stabilize the jaw on the opposite side of the stimulus)
Bilateral Tongue Hugs	Any age 1+		Lingual elongation	2 Z-Vibes® with small green square heads
Pre-feeding Chewing Hierarchy 1	4-6 months and up		Symmetrical chew Tongue retraction Lateral chew	Yellow and/or red Chewy Tubes® Z-Vibe® preefer tip Trimmed toothette

A Sensory Motor Approach to Feeding

Utensils/Size and Shape of Food/Placement of Food:

Use a side spoon placement to provoke lip closure.	
Cut all foods into cube size portions that are big enough to feel yet small enough to handle.	
Placement of Food	Food should be placed on the lateral molar ridge about where the first molar is located. Place the cube on the molar ridge (B) and provide slight downward pressure to facilitate a munch chew
Solid Utensil - Cocktail fork/Narrow Fork	
Cup Drinking - use recessed lid cup	
Straw Drinking - resolve tongue thrusting and exaggerated tongue protrusion with Honey Bear Straw Cup	

Chapter 10: Writing a Program Plan

HOME BASE	ONE CHANGE	⟶	NEW FOOD
Mac and Cheese	Taste	Add new shredded cheese to recipe	Variety of mac and cheese flavors
Peanut Butter	Texture	Buy chunky variety	Chunky peanut butter
	Taste	Almond	Almond butter
	Temperature	Freeze	Peanut butter "ball"
Bread	Texture	Toast	Crunchy bread
	Taste	Add hummus	Bread with hummus
	Taste	Add olive oil spread	Bread dipped into good fat
	Taste	Pan fry with egg and butter	French toast
Chicken Nuggets	Texture	Oven baked as opposed to fried	Same item new texture
	Taste	Dip in mayo to add fat/calories	Same item new flavor
	Texture	Make with panko bread crumbs	Accept new type of nugget
Chicken Leg	Texture	Broil chicken	Crispier skin, if he will eat- adds fat
	Taste	Stew in red sauce	Try to add pasta to the meal as well
French Fries	Taste	Use yams or sweet potatoes	Sweet potato fries
Juice	Taste	Use mango nectar and other orange-colored juices	Mango nectar, Peach nectar
	Texture	Blend with ice and Greek yogurt for protein	Smoothie

A Sensory Motor Approach to Feeding

CASE #3: JOHN

PROGRAM PLAN

Sensory/Pre-Feeding:

This plan should be implemented 2-3 times per day.

The goal of a pre-feeding program is to develop the motor skills to support safe, effective, nutritive feeding. John's plan should be implemented 2-3 times per day. The plan should be done in conjunction with whole body sensory input. John will benefit from being in a well supported seated position with his hips at a 90-degree angle, knees at a 90-degree angle, and feet grounded.

1. **Massage:** Start at the temporomandibular joint (TMJ) and provide firm, elongated massage to the corners of John's lips, alongside the nostrils into the insertion of the upper lip, and from under the nostrils into the upper lip. Do each set 4-5 times. Vary the sensory input and incorporate into daily living activities.

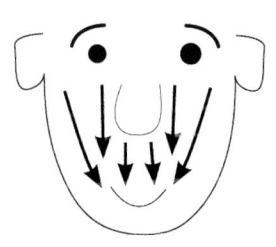

Sensory Suggestions:

- Bare hands – prior to meals, play
- Lotion – after bath
- Wet/dry washcloths – before/after meals, after bath
- Warm/cold washcloths – bath time
- Textured bean bags – play
- Vibration – play

This will increase sensory awareness and organization, encourage midline orientation and facilitate increased cheek and upper lip mobility.

2. **Tap-n-Tone:** Provide firm, rhythmic tapping from the TMJ to the corners of the lips and on the surface of the lips to the beat of a favorite finger play activity or nursery rhyme.

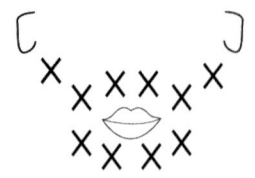

This will provide sensory input and tone the buccal and labial musculature.

3. **Cheek Stretch:** Present the Z-vibe® yellow head or iced, trimmed toothette in his cheek. Stroke the inside of his cheek from top to bottom 4-5 times on one side. Repeat on the opposite side.

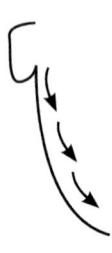

This will increase sensory awareness and mobility through the buccal musculature.

4. **Lateral Tongue Massage:** Stroke the lateral borders of the tongue from back to front 4-5 times on one side and then 4-5 times on the opposite side. This can be done with the Z-Vibe® yellow head or a trimmed toothette dipped in cold water.

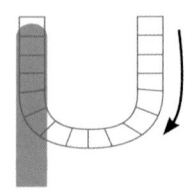

This will provide sensory information and elongation through the lateral borders of the tongue.

5. **Cheek Toning/Lip Rounding:** Present the rounded end of the Jiggler between John's lips. Provide jaw/cheek support as needed to facilitate lip rounding. Repeat 10 times or as John will tolerate.

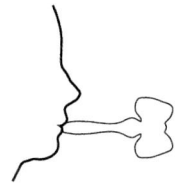

This will provide sensory input, facilitate increased tone in the cheeks, and encourage lip rounding.

5. **Alternating Chewy Tubes:**

   1. Present a yellow chewy tube perpendicular to the lateral molar ridge at John's first molar.

   2. Quickly present a second yellow chewy tube on the opposite molar ridge.

   3. Alternate biting on one side and then the other for 10 repetitions.

   4. Work towards 2 bites on each side. Goal: 5 graded, repetitive bites on each side.

Feeding:

   1. **Spoon Feeding:** Use a flat-bowled spoon for purees. Turn the spoon sideways, contacting the corners of John's lips. Tilt the spoon slightly if you observe him biting the spoon.

This will encourage lip closure and tongue retraction.

   2. **Straw Drinking:** John should be drinking from TalkTools® straw #1. Over the next several weeks soak the top of the straw in hot water and

trim above the character. Eventually there should only be ¼ inch of straw above the character.

This will increase lip rounding and tongue retraction.

3. **Chewing Hierarchy:** Follow the directions on the protocol for Chewing Hierarchy Level #1 using ice straws or stuffed chewy tubes. Alternate sides and repeat.

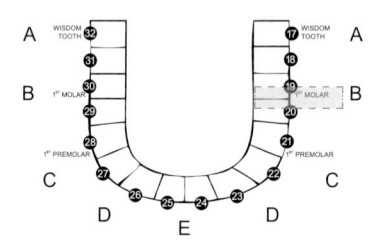

This will encourage a lateral chew, jaw grading, and tongue retraction.

Re-evaluation: Four months.

Additional Information:

Music to support motor planning and a Spio garment are recommended supports.

        www.expresstrain.org
        www.spioworks.com

6) Goals and Objectives

School systems and insurance companies require goals and objectives that are individualized for each child. Different school systems and insurance companies require different formats. Goals and objectives help both therapists, and non-therapists (parents, doctors, teachers, etc.) monitor progress.

Sara Rosenfeld-Johnson and Robyn Merkel-Walsh of TalkTools® created

Oral Placement Therapy Goals and *Objectives for IEPs* and *Insurance Reimbursement.* This CD was designed to help therapists write accurate IEP goals, in order to accurately measure progress in Oral Placement Therapy (OPT) activities used to improve feeding and speech clarity. This CD Rom includes both feeding and speech goals, but for the purpose of this text, we have adapted the goals and objectives to coincide with the previous feeding program plans. Example goals and objectives include:

CASE #1: SEAN

Goal: Sean will improve pre-feeding skills to support safe, nutritive feedings.

Objectives:

- Will tolerate the SLP touching the face
- Will increase sensory awareness and organization
- Will increase midline orientation
- Will increase tone in the buccal and labial musculature
- Will increase upper lip mobility
- Will increase lip rounding
- Will increase jaw strength
- Will increase tongue retraction
- Will improve jaw grading
- Will improve jaw/lip dissociation

CASE #2: JOE

Goal: Joe will improve pre-feeding skills to support safe, nutritive feedings.

Objectives:

- Will improve cheek mobility
- Will improve lip mobility
- Will decrease use of a bottle

- Will increase use of a straw
- Will tolerate intra-oral stimulation
- Will achieve a 75% retraction to 25% protrusion tongue posture
- Will eliminate tongue thrusting
- Will transfer bolus across midline
- Will tolerate a variety of tastes, temperatures, and textures

CASE #3: JOHN

Goal: John will improve pre-feeding skills to support safe, nutritive feedings.

Objectives:

- Will increase sensory awareness
- Will increase cheek mobility
- Will increase upper lip mobility
- Will elongate the lateral borders of the tongue
- Will improve lip rounding
- Will improve lip closure
- Will improve tongue retraction
- Will improve lip rounding
- Will improve jaw/lip/tongue dissociation

CONCLUSION:

When conducting a pre–feeding and feeding assessment, it is critical to write a report that not only includes a diagnosis, but outlines goals, objectives, and activities desirable for facilitating safe nutritive feedings. There will be six sections of each report: 1) Identifying data; 2) Background Information; 3) Testing Observations; 4) Summary and Recommendations; 5) Program Plan; and 6) Goals and Objectives. Various writing styles may be used; however the content of the report should always include the aforementioned information. This chapter has outlined the writing process involved in thorough report writing. For a full report example, please refer to Appendix E.

APPENDIX A:
GLUTEN-FREE, CASEIN-FREE DIET

Gluten, a protein rich in amino acids, is found in wheat. Casein is a protein found in cow's milk. These two proteins have been linked to allergies and gastrointestinal diseases including Leaky Gut Syndrome , GERD, and constipation (Hassal, 2005).

Over the past ten years, the general public has paid more attention to gluten and dairy sensitivities than ever before. As many as eighteen million people world-wide have gluten sensitivities and/or Celiac Disease. Some researchers believe that all humans have gluten intolerance to some degree, and this is not a protein that was meant for human digestion (Fasano, 2011).

In the field of Autism especially, studies have concluded that Gluten/Casein Free Diets are preferable for children on the spectrum (Balzola et al., 2006). As mentioned in Chapter 4, Defeat Autism Now suggests that a GFCF Diet be followed.

With consideration of these issues, TalkTools® Instructors are careful in considering the types of food we use in our Program Plans. When choosing food types for therapeutic feeding, it is helpful to use GFCF products, especially with children who have a diagnosis of Autism Spectrum Disorder (Merkel-Walsh, 2012).

Always check the label and make sure it is GF Certified and/or has a Kosher Parve label. Kosher Parve labels indicate that the product is dairy free, not that it is gluten free.

Food Type	GFCF Alternative
Cubed Solids	Del Monte® Canned Vegetables
	Galaxy® Nutritional Foods cheeses
	Kellogg's® Corn Pops Cereal
	Health Valley® Rice Checks cereal
	Starburst® Fruit Chews
	Skittles®
	Mother's® Rice Cakes
	Bionaturae® Organic Gluten Free Pasta
	Bell and Evans® Gluten-Free Chicken Nuggets
	Nature's Path® Gorilla Munch Cereal
	Kitov® Corn Pops (Kosher)
	Cantaloupe, Honey Dew and Watermelon
	Tinkayda® Brown Rice Pasta, Elbows or Penne
	Seedless Cucumber, Peeled
	Glutino® Bread
	Frookie® Cookies
	Robert's American Gourmet® Potato Flyers
	Van's® Wheat-Gluten Free Waffles
	Quaker® Mini Rice Cakes
	Ian's® Allergy Friendly Chicken Nuggets and Fish Sticks
	Muncho's® Potato Chips
	Crunchmaster® Crackers
	Quinoa® Pasta
Strip Feeding	Van's® Wheat-Gluten Free Waffles
	Ore-Ida® Cottage Fries
	McCain's® 5-Minute Fries
	Alexis® Sweet Potato Fries
	Ian's® Allergy Friendly Fish Sticks
	Stretch Island® Fruit Leather
	Applegate Farms® Chicken and Turkey Hot Dogs (Nitrate Free)
	Applegate Farms® Oven-Roasted Turkey Breast
	Applegate Farms® Chicken and Apple Breakfast Sausage
	Bakery On® Main Granola Bars
	Real Foods® Corn Thins
	Arrowhead® Gluten Free Baking Mix (to make pancakes or waffles)
	Schar® Gluten-Free Ladyfingers
	Snikiddy® All Natural Baked Fries
	Glutino® Gluten-Free Pretzels
	Dr. Praeger's® Little Broccoli and Potato "Patties"

Puree for Spoon Feeding	Imagine Foods® Pudding
	SO Delicious® Dairy Free Coconut Milk Yogurt
	Rice Dream® Ice Cream
	Frito Lay® Burrito
	Frito Lay® Bean Dip
	Dole® Fruit Sorbet
	Edy's® Whole Fruit Sorbet
	Mott's® Plain Applesauce (watch for Calcium Lactate Additives in many apple sauces)
	Earth's Best® Stage 1-2 Fruits (Check each jar some contain wheat and milk)
	Ortega® Salsa
	Hip Whip® Non-Dairy Topping
	Red Mill® Oats
	Happy Baby® Frozen Organic Baby Foods
Calorie Activities	Neocate® Nutra
	Neocate® Splash
	Rice Flakes
	Quinoa® Flakes
	Flaxseed Oil

APPENDIX B:
THE ORAL SENSORY-MOTOR COOKBOOK FOOD SUGGESTIONS

1. *Formula*
    - Premature (Similac®, Enfamil®)
    - Postdischarge - Similac® (Neosure), Enfamil® (Enfacare)
    - Cow's Milk Based - Enfamil®, Similac,® Store Brand, Bright Beginnings®
    - Soy Based - Enfamil® (Prosobee), Similac® (Isomil), Bright Beginnings®, Gerber® (Good Start) *Note:* Based on currently available research soy formulas should only be used if recommended by a physician.
    - Hydrolyzed Whey Based - Gerber® (Good Start)
    - Hydrolyzed Casein Based - Similac® (Alimentum), Enfamil® (Nutramigen)
    - Hydrolyzed Casein/Whey Based - Enfamil® (Gentlease)
    - Amino Acid (Elemental) Based - Nutricia North America® (Neocate), Abbott Nutrition® (Elecare)

2. *Spoon Feeding*

    Homemade baby food is recommended and can be pureed to Stage I consistency in blenders such as the "bullet" food processor, Beaba Babycook® (Williams-Sonoma) or Baby Brezza® (Williams-Sonoma).

    Happy Baby pouches are recommended for commercially available baby foods.

A. **Smooth Purees:**
- Sweet Potatoes
- Carrots
- Zucchini
- Squash, Butternut Squash
- Asparagus
- Beets
- Bananas
- Applesauce
- Plums
- Apricots
- Pears
- Kiwi
- Mango
- Nectarines
- Avocado
- Spinach
- Yogurt

B. **Cereals:**
- Rice
- Oat
- Barley

C. **Textured Purees:**
- Rice
- Quinoa
- Beans
- Hummus
- Broccoli
- Cauliflower
- Yogurt with Fruit
- Mixed Baby Foods

D. Pureed Meats:
    Chicken
    Turkey
    Beef
    Meat and Vegetable Combinations
    Meat and Quinoa, Rice or Pasta Combinations

- Suggestions for the Low Tone Toddler
    Cinnamon Flavored Applesauce
    Frozen Fruit Purees
    Garlic Humus
    Baba Ganoush with Tahini (if no allergies to seeds)
    Ground "Table" Foods
    Guacamole
    Puree of Minestrone Soup
    Yogurt: Lemon, Coffee

3. *Cubed Solids*
    Gerber® Stars, Puffs
    Veggie Booty®
    Cheerios®
    Cubed Waffles, Pancakes, French Toast
    Avocado Cubes
    Potato Or Sweet Potato Cubes
    Carrots (cooked and cubed)
    Beets (cooked and cubed)
    Banana (cubed)
    Melon (cubed)
    Apple or Pear (baked and cubed)
    Skinned/Cubed Turkey, Chicken or Beef Hot Dogs
    Matzoh Balls, Potato Pancakes (cubed)
    Meatballs (make them soft with extra bread crumbs) (cubed)
    Chicken Nuggets (cubed)
    Fish Sticks (cubed)

Rotisserie Chicken (cubed)
Pasta
Cubes of Cheese

4. *Strips*

Veggie Stix® Snacks
French Fries
Chicken Tender Strips
Luncheon Meats (cut into chunks and then strip shapes)
Twice-Grilled Cheese Sandwiches
Grilled Cheese and Potato Chip Sandwiches
Waffle Strips
Hamburger Strips
Pizza Bagel Strips
Barilla® Pasta (gemelli, long ziti noodles)
Steamed Carrot Sticks (dipped in salad dressing or vinegar)
Pickle Spears
Thin Pretzel Sticks
Cheetos®
Bambas®
Apple Slices
Steamed String Beans
Jicama Sticks
Daikon Sticks

Kosher options:
Veggie Fries®
Veggie Straws®
Keffli
Bambas®
"Pea Pods"

5. *Suggestions for Adding Sensory Input to Food (taste)*
　　Cinnamon
　　Nutmeg
　　Allspice
　　Garlic Powder
　　Vinegar
　　Seasoned Salt
　　Pepper
　　Teriyaki Sauce
　　Ketchup
　　Sautéed Fresh Garlic
　　Curry
　　Salsa
　　Extracts
　　Salad Dressings
　　Fresh Herbs: Parsley, Oregano, Thyme, Rosemary, Basil
　　Sparkling Water (plain or mixed with any juice)

6. *Suggestions for Adding Texture*

   Note: There are some contraindications to using commercially available thickeners and rice cereal. Check with your physician before choosing a thickener.

　　Baby food thinned with spring water (this is preferred for babies under a year of age starting cup drinking with thickened liquid.)
　　Nectar rather than Juice
　　Rice Cereal
　　Thik & Clear® Food Thickener or Simply Thick®
　　Wheat Germ
　　Flax Seed
　　Ground Crackers or Graham Crackers

7. Low Tone Drink Suggestions

Note: Juice is "empty calories". For children with compromised nutrition avoid sugary fruit juice.

- Lemonade
- Limeade
- Grapefruit
- Cranberry
- Tamarind
- Orange Juice
- Mango or Papaya Nectar
- Gatorade®
- Smoothies (fruit or vegetable)

8. Suggestions to Add Calories

Note: A registered dietitian, nutritionist, or physician should be consulted before adding caloric boosters.

- MCT Oil
- Polycose Powder
- Beneprotein
- Scandical Powder (by Scandipharm®)
- Microlipid®
- Benecalorie (by Nestle®)
- Duocal® Super Soluble Powder
- Vegetable Oil, Olive Oil
- Powdered Milk, Condensed Milk
- Half and Half to Milk (if there are no dairy intolerances)
- Butter
- Peanut Butter, Soy Nut Butter
- Pureed Beans, Avocado
- Half and Half to Milk

9. Examples of Calorie Supplements:
- Pediasure®
- Boost® (Boost Breeze)
- Ensure® (pudding)
- Ultracare® for Kids

10. Foods to Avoid for GERD *(if symptoms worsen with these foods)*
- Citrus
- Tomato
- Vinegar
- Peppermint
- Fatty Food
- Carbonation
- Chocolate
- Caffeine
- Ketchup
- Spicy Food

Note: See Gluten Free/Casein Free suggestions for clients who have intolerances to these foods.

APPENDIX C:
NUTRITIONAL GUIDELINES

MyPyramid Suggested Calories & Intake Amounts for Children Ages 2 to 18 Years*

Food Group	Age 2-3 Years 1000-1400 Calories**	Age 4-8 Years 1200-2000 Calories**	Age 9-13 Years 1600-2600 Calories**	Age 14-18 Years 2000-3200 Calories**
Fruits	1 cup to 1.5 cups	1 cup to 2 cups	1.5 cups to 2 cups	2 cups to 2.5 cups
	Fresh, frozen, canned, dried fruit and fruit juices. 1 cup fruit or 100% juice or ½ cup dried fruit = 1 cup			
Vegetables	1 cup to 1.5 cups	1.5 cups to 2.5 cups	2 cups to 3.5 cups	2.5 cups to 4 cups
	Fresh, frozen, canned, dried vegetable and vegetable juices. Dark green, orange, legumes, starchy and other vegetables have specific recommendations.† 1 cup raw, cooked vegetable or vegetable juice or 2 cups raw leafy greens = 1 cup.			
Grains	3 oz-eq to 5 oz eq	4 oz eq to 6 oz eq	5 oz eq to 9 oz eq	6 oz eq to 10 oz eq
	All foods made from rice, oats, barley, wheat, including bread, pasta, oatmeal, cereals, and crackers. 1 slice bread, 1 cup dry cereal, ½ cup cooked rice, cereal or pasta = 1 oz equivalent. At least half of all grains should be whole grains.			
Milk	2 cups	2 cups to 3 cups	3 cups	3 cups
	All fluid milk and products made from milk. Does not include cream and butter. 1 cup milk or yogurt, 1.5 oz natural cheese, 2 oz processed cheese = 1 cup			
Meat & Beans	2 oz eq to 4 oz eq	3 oz eq to 5.5 oz eq	5 oz eq to 6.5 oz eq	5.5 oz eq to 7 oz eq
	1 oz lean meat, fish, poultry, 1 egg, 1 Tbsp. peanut butter, ¼ cup cooked dry beans, ½ oz nuts = 1 oz equivalent			
Oils	3 tsp to 4 tsp	4 tsp to 6 tsp	5 tsp to 8 tsp	6 tsp to 11 tsp
	Sources such as corn, safflower, sunflower, canola, corn, olive oils, as well as some nuts, fish, avocados, mayonnaise, salad dressings and margarine			

*Recommendations will vary within stated ranges for males, females and ages. Please refer to www.MyPyramid.gov for detailed recommendations.
**Based on activity levels of 'Sedentary' < 30 minutes per day, 'Mod Active' 30-60 minutes per day, and 'Active' > 60 minutes per day, and calculations for Estimated Energy Requirements (EER) from the Institute of Medicine.
†Vegetable subgroup amounts per week can be found at www.MyPyramid.gov.

Source: United States Department of Agriculture Center for Nutrition Policy and Promotion.

APPENDIX D:
FORMS

ORAL-MOTOR/FEEDING EVALUATION CHECKLIST A

Name:

D.O.B.:
D.O.E.:

Diagnosis:

+ = Observed
− = Not Observed

Tone

__ Low
__ High
__ Mixed

Palate

__ Intact
__ High Vault
__ Flat
__ Ridgy

Dentition

__ Normal Bite (Class I)
__ Under Bite (Class II)
__ Over Bite (Class III)
__ Cross Bite
__ Open Bite (Over Jet)
__ Diastemas (Spaces Between Teeth)
__ Misplaced Teeth _____

Velopharyngeal closure

__ Adequate   __ Inadequate

	Structure	**Functions**
Labial (lips)	Cleft	Closure
	Symmetry	Opening
	Shape/Size	Retraction
		Rounding
		Dissociating
		Grading
Lingual (tongue)	Heart-Shaped Tip	Retraction
	Asymmetry	Protrusion
	Bulging	Lateralization
	Deep Midline	Tongue-Tip Pointing
	Lingual Frenum	Tongue-Tip Elevation
		Tongue-Tip Depression
Jaw	Small/Retracted	Stability
	Protruded	Dissociation (rotary movement)
	Asymmetry	Grading
Cheeks	Tone	Stability
	Symmetry	Movement

Oral Habits:

Teeth Grinding
Thumb Sucking
Mouth Breathing
Mouthing Objects
Spitting
Digit Sucking

Diet Summary:

Texture:

Taste:

Temperature:

Size/Shape:

Evaluation Checklist Form B

WNL	Within Normal Limits	**NA**	Not Applicable	**R**	Remarkable
+T	Hypertonia	**H**	History Of	**-D**	Poor Dissociation
S	Severely Impaired	**-T**	Hypotonia	**O**	Observed

1. Hard Tissue

BONE STRUCTURE		SIDE PROFILE	
Mesocephalic (normal)		Straight	
Dolicocephalic (narrow angles)		Convex	
Brachycephalic (wide angles)		Concave	
Symmetrical		High Nasio-Labial Angle	
Asymmetrical			
High palate			
Wide palate			
Narrow palate			
Flat palate			
Clefting			

2. Jaw/Dentition

Class I		Open Bite	
Class II		Indentia/Spacing	
Class III		Loose Teeth	
Overbite		Missing Teeth	
Underbite		Crowding	
Overjet		Crossbite	
Orthodontics		Jaw Grading	
		Jaw Stability	

3. Soft Tissue

Soft Palate		Tongue	
Lips		Buccal Muscles	
Uvula		Tonsils and Adenoids	
Thrust		Mouth Ulcers	
Sublabia Frenum		Sublingual Frenum	
Nursing Pads			

4. Oral Habits/Oral Resting Postures

Teeth Grinding		Spitting	
Thumb Sucking		Digit Sucking	
Mouthing Objects		Jaw Tensing	
Open-Mouth Posture		Nose Breather	
Mouth Breather		Mixed Breathing	
Chronic Anterior Tongue Posture		Drooling	

5. Sensory

Defensive		Seeking Oral Input	
Tolerates Massage		Tolerates Vibration	
Tolerates Textures		Reacts to Smell	
Visual Sensitivity		Sensitivity to Sound	
Self Stimulatory Behaviors		Has a Sensory Diet	

Comments:

6. Coordination and Dissociation

JAW		LIPS		TONGUE	
Stability		Protrusion		Protrusion	
Grading		Rounding		Retraction	
		Closure		Lateralization	
		Retraction		Elevation	
		Sequential Mvmt.		Sequential Mvt.	

7. Feeding

Defensive to Various Foods		Has a Good Diet	
Gag Reflex		Munch Chewing	
Prolonged Bottle Use		Pacifier	
Used Sippy Cup for more than 3-6 Months		Rotary Chew Developed	
Can Lateralize Bolus Across The Midline		Straw Drinking	
Cup Drinking		Tongue Thrust	

Case History Information Form A
Feeding Evaluation

Date: _____

Name: _____ DOB: _____

Address: _____ Age: _____
        _____ Daytime Phone: _____
        _____ Other Phone: _____

Referral Source: _____

What is your concern about your child's feeding? Has the condition changed in the past six months?

SchoolPlacement:_____

Classification:_____

Current Services:

PT _____ OT: _____ ST:_____

Pediatrician's Name and Address (to mail report):

I. FAMILY HISTORY

Mother's Name _____ Age _____

Occupation _____ Place of Birth_____

Father's Name _____ Age _____

Occupation _____ Place of Birth_____

Who lives in the home?

Name_____ Age _____ Relationship _____

What languages are spoken at home?

Are there any speech and language difficulties?

Have any other specialists seen the child?

II. BIRTH HISTORY

Length of pregnancy: _____weeks. Did you smoke cigarettes, drink alcoholic beverages, take medication or use drugs during your pregnancy?

Were there any complications during pregnancy? If so, please explain.

Were there any problems during labor and delivery? If so, please explain. Was delivery vaginal or by caesarean section?

What was the child's weight and general condition at birth?

III. MEDICAL HISTORY

Has your child been hospitalized? If so, include age, reason, and length of stay.

History of illness, including age.

History of accidents, including age.

How would you describe your child's general health?

Does your child have allergies or frequent colds? If so, describe.

Is your child currently under a doctor's care? Is s/he taking any medication? If so, what kind and why?

Has your child's hearing been tested? If so, when and what are the results? Does your child have a history of middle ear infections? If so, include when and how often. Has he/she required ear surgery?

Has your child's vision been tested? What were the results?

IV. DEVELOPMENTAL HISTORY

At what age did your child:

roll over_____   stand independently_____
sit independently_____   walk independently_____
crawl _____   toilet train_____
finger feed_____   self-feed with utensils_____
first vocalize_____   babble_____
ay first words_____   combine words_____
talk in complete sentences_____

Oral/Feeding Habits and Sensory Information
(Has your child had any feeding difficulties? (e.g., drooling, swallowing) Does he/she avoid any foods?)

When did your child wean from a bottle?

Did your child use a Sippy Cup for more than 3-6 months?
Does your child use a straw to drink liquids?

When did your child stop sucking his/her thumb or digits?

Did your child use a pacifier? If so, for how long?

Does your child grind his teeth/or tense his jaw?

Does your child exhibit open mouth posture and mouth breathe?

Is your child sensitive to textures?

Is your child sensitive to sounds?

Is your child sensitive to smell?

Is your child tactile defensive?

Does your child exhibit any self stimulatory behaviors? If so describe.

Which hand does your child use primarily?

Does your child seem to have any balance or coordination difficulties? If so, please describe.

How are your child's sleeping patterns?

How does your child currently communicate his/her wants and needs?

How clear is your child's speech?

How well does your child understand what is being said to him/her?

V. SOCIAL HISTORY

How would you describe your child's personality?

Describe your child's socialization skills with family and familiar people.

How does your child react to unfamiliar people and/or situations?

How does your child interact with other children?

What are your child's favorite activities/hobbies?

Describe your child's activity level.

VI. ADDITIONAL INFORMATION

Is there any other information about your child that would be helpful to us in evaluating your child ? Please explain.

Please list the name brand of your child's utensils, cups, straws, and/or bottles that are being used at this time:

Please describe how your child is positioned during feedings, including where the child sits, what is happening around the child, and how long it takes the child to eat:

If possible, please provide photos of your child at mealtimes.
Videos would also be appreciated.

Case History Information Form B
Feeding Evaluation

Client's Name: _____

Address: _____

City: _____ State: _____ Zip: _____

Phone: (Home) _____ (Work) _____ (Cell) _____

Birth Date: _____ Age: _____

Parents' Names: _____ Email: _____

Predominant Language Spoken in Home: _____

**VIDEOTAPING: I give my permission for the Evaluation to be videotaped for educational purposes.

Parent Signature _____ Date _____

I. FAMILY HISTORY

Child lives with: Both Parents _____   Mother _____

Father _____   Other: _____

Names and ages of brothers and sisters:
_____

_____

Is there any history of speech, language, hearing problems, learning issues, or delays in other family members? If so, please describe:
_____

_____

II. BIRTH HISTORY

Did you have any problems during pregnancy? Yes _____ No _____
Please describe: _____

_____

Did you carry this baby full term? Yes _____ No _____
If no, indicate length of pregnancy in weeks: _____

Were there any problems with the delivery? Yes _____ No _____
Please describe: _____

_____

Did your baby require any special care after delivery? _____

_____

What was the baby's weight at birth? _____ Apgar scores? _____

III. MEDICAL HISTORY

Does your child have a diagnosis (i.e., birth defect, genetic disorder, development delay)? _____

_____

Does your child have any of the following:

____ Frequent Colds/Upper Respiratory Disorders
____ Frequent Strep Throat/Sore Throat
____ Recurrent Middle Ear Infections
____ Asthma
____ Heart Condition
____ Kidney Issues or Urinary Issues
____ Vision Issues
____ GI Issues

____ Constipation   ____ Reflux
____ Diarrhea   ____ Failure To Thrive

____ Allergies
____ Seizures

Has your child ever been hospitalized? If so, please describe:
_____

Has your child ever had surgery? If so, please explain:
_____

Does your child have difficulty hearing? Yes _____ No _____

Has the hearing been tested? Yes _____ No _____

What are the results of the hearing test? _____

Is your child taking any medications on a regular basis? Yes _____ No _____
If yes, please list the medications and reasons child is taking them:

_____

Please list the names and addresses of all of the physicians and therapists who care for your child:

_____
_____
_____

IV. DEVELOPMENTAL HISTORY

Milestones: List the approximate age when your child first began to:

Hold Head Up _____ Roll Over _____ Sit Alone _____

Crawl _____ Stand Independently _____

Walk _____ Reach for Objects _____

Cross Midline with an Object _____

Show a Hand Preference _____

Spoon Feed Independently _____

Toilet Train _____ Dress Self _____

Babble and Coo _____

Speak in Jargon _____

Use Single Words _____

Combine 2 Words _____ 3 or More Words _____

V. FEEDING ISSUES

Do you or your physician have any concerns about your child's nutritional status? Yes ____ No ____ Please explain: _____

Do you or your physician have concerns about safety issues related to oral feeding? _____

What is your child's current height/weight? _____

Was your child breast fed _____ or bottle fed _____ ?

Did your child have any difficulties nursing or bottle feeding (i.e., crying, gagging, coughing, reflux, difficulty latching on)? Yes ____ No ____ Please explain: _____

At what age did you introduce spoon feeding? _____
Did your child have any difficulty with pureed foods? Yes ____ No ____
Please explain: _____

At what age did you introduce solid foods (i.e., Cheerios)? _____

Did your child have any difficulties with solids? Yes ____ No ____
Please explain: _____

Is your child on a restrictive diet (i.e., Gluten Free, etc.)?
_____

Does your child have any food aversions? Yes ____ No ____
Please explain:
____ Taste (i.e., sweet, salty, spicy): _____

____ Texture (pureed, soft solids, chewy, crunchy): _____

___ Temperature (warm, cold, room temperature): _____

___ Color: _____

___ Size/Shape: _____

Does your child have any unusual food preferences?
_____

If your child is tube fed please answer the following:

Is your child OG, NG, or G-tube fed? _____

Is your child bolus fed (by hand) or on a continuous drip (pump)?
(over what time period?) _____
_____

Please note the amount of food, what type of formula or blended foods are used. Please record a five-day baseline diet:

	DAY 1	DAY 2	DAY 3	DAY 4	DAY 5
BREAKFAST					
LUNCH					
DINNER					
SNACK					

VI. SENSORY ISSUES

Does your child have any of the following issues?

___ Get upset easily
___ Have difficulty calming
___ Have difficulty sitting still
___ Experience more than normal separation issues
___ Have sleeping issues
___ Have eating issues
___ Have attention issues
___ Have difficulty transitioning from one activity to another
___ Perseverate on objects or activities
___ Have complicated routines for bed, bath, mealtime, etc.
___ Cover his/her ears in response to otherwise typical sounds/noises
___ Have difficulty with daily living activities (tooth brushing, hair washing, etc.)
___ Dislike having their hands dirty

VII. SOCIAL HISTORY

What are your child's play preferences? _____

Does your child attend Nursery School and/or regular group activities with other children? Yes _____   No _____
If yes, where? _____

How does your child relate to other children?
_____
_____
_____

What comments have other adults, e.g., teachers, made about your child's speech and language?
_____
_____
_____

Compared to other children of similar age, how would you describe your child's overall behaviors and ability to listen and follow directions?

_____
_____
_____

VIII. SCHOOLING

Present School Placement: _____

Address: _____
_____

Telephone: _____

Type of Therapy (Speech, O.T., P.T.): _____

Therapist's Name: _____

IX. CONCERNS

In your own words, please describe your concerns about your child's oral motor, feeding, speech or language abilities.

_____
_____
_____

X. REFERRED BY

_____
Name   Telephone

_____
Client/Parent Signature   Date

5 Day Baseline Diet

	1	2	3	4	5
BREAKFAST					
LUNCH					
SNACK					
DINNER					
SNACK					
ADDITIONAL NOTES					

Home Base:

Texture -

Temperature -

Taste -

APPENDIX E:
SAMPLE REPORT

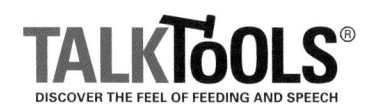

TALKTOOLS®
DISCOVER THE FEEL OF FEEDING AND SPEECH

Name: Sean Martin	DOB: 1/1/08
Address: 32 Main Street City, State Zip	Chronological Age: 3.11
Phone: 201.555.1211	Parents Names: Sean and Maria Martin
Primary Physician: Dr. Kim	Referring Physician: Dr. Kim
Diagnosis: bilateral open-lip schizencephaly and right hemiparesis	Procedure Code: 92610

BACKGROUND INFORMATION:

Sean, a 3.11-year-old boy with a diagnosis of bilateral open lip schizencephaly/right hemiparesis was seen for an oral motor/feeding evaluation. Sean was accompanied by his mother and grandparents, who served as informants. Sean was referred for this evaluation by Dr. Kim, secondary to concerns about safe, nutritive feeding.

Sean is the product of a full term pregnancy and uncomplicated delivery. Neonatal course was reportedly uneventful. Early motor development was a concern, and at 10 months of age, Sean was diagnosed with bilateral open lip schizencephaly and right hemiparesis. Medical history is significant for constipation. Sean has had Botox treatments on his right arm and leg which have yielded positive results with mobility. More recently, he had Botox treatments on his salivary glands to decrease drooling. However, there have not been notable changes in saliva control.

Sean was successfully bottle-fed and transitioned to purees without incident. He reportedly has always been a messy eater and loses food on the right side of his mouth. Sean's solid foods are limited by his mother and grandparents secondary to safety concerns. Soft solids are cut into very small pieces as Sean "does not really chew well." Raw vegetables, meat, crunchy snacks (chips), hard fruit, and bagels, are difficult for Sean. He drinks from an open cup and a straw. He is more successful with a toddler sippy cup. To date, he has not had a specific pre-feeding program. His family has been told to "rub a Z-vibe® on his face and in his mouth" prior to feeding.

DISCUSSION:

Sean's evaluation and summary were recorded on video for his family and team. The following is an overview of the clinical observations:

- Sean presented with posture and muscle tone issues which impacted feeding and speech. He had shortened pectoralis muscles, decreased rib cage mobility, flared ribs, and decreased abdominal/oblique support for controlled respiration. Respiration was shallow and did not support more than one or two words at a time. Tone in the oral musculature was reduced, but movement patterns in the lips and tongue reflect extensor patterns.

- Sean had a high palatal vault.

- Sean's jaw symmetry, strength, and stability were notably compromised. Jaw sliding was observed at rest. A non-dissociated, poorly graded munch chew (with food forward in the oral cavity) was observed with all textures. Wide jaw excursions were noted with chewing, sucking on a sippy cup nipple, and sound production. Sean does not have adequate strength to masticate a solid bolus, and he often swallowed food that was not adequately broken down/chewed. There was no evidence of emerging jaw/lip/tongue dissociation or grading for feeding or sound production.

- The buccal musculature was poorly defined, and Sean did not use his cheeks to support sucking, chewing, swallowing, stabilizing a solid bolus, or sound production.

- The labial musculature was retracted at rest and during support function. Sean did not have functional bilateral approximation for spoon feeding. He bit the spoon and cleared the bolus with a non-dissociated trunk, shoulder, neck, jaw movement. He did not approximate lip closure during chewing. Labial seal on a straw or cup was poor (particularly on the right side), and Sean compensated by using his tongue.

- The lingual musculature was bulgy and poorly defined. Sean did not use the lateral borders of his tongue or tongue tip functionally. Sean's primary lingual movement continued to be a suckle (protrusion/retraction). He used this pattern along with tongue dumping to move a solid bolus. Food is transported to the canine (not the first molar) for mastication. Food fell onto the lingual surface and was suckled at midline. The bolus was handled in the front third of the mouth and was often spread across the tongue.

- With regard to sensory processing, Sean clearly had reduced awareness both inside and outside of the mouth. He was a copious drooler and is seemingly unaware of saliva running down his chin. He stuffed his mouth, and sought salty high-taste foods. Sean frequently did not clear a solid bolus and residual food pooled on the lateral borders of the tongue and within his palate. Sean also "stopped chewing" with residual food in his mouth and appeared to be unaware of food held intra-orally.

- Sean took a long time to break down food and often swallowed a poorly masticated bolus. This presented a significant choking risk.

SUMMARY:

Sean presents with neuro-motor, muscle tone, and oral sensory-motor issues which clearly impact both feeding and speech. He has made great gains in gross and fine motor development. Significant challenges persist in both feeding and speech sound production.

The following program plan was developed to address the development of oral sensory-motor skills to support safe, effective, nutritive feeding.

I would be happy to work with Sean's family and team as this plan is implemented. I can best be reached via email at feedingslp@123.com. Sean's mother and grandmother will update me periodically via email. I would like to re-evaluate Sean in approximately four months to assess his progress and update his plan.

DIAGNOSIS:
(783.3) Feeding Mismanagement
(784.51) Oral Facial Hypotonia

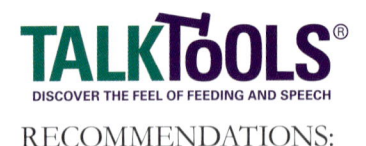

RECOMMENDATIONS:

Oral Sensory-Motor Feeding Therapy twice weekly by a speech-language pathologist with post-graduate training in feeding disorders.

Sensory/Pre-Feeding: This plan should be implemented 2-3 times per day.

GOALS: Sean will improve pre-feeding skills to support safe, nutritive feedings.

Objectives:

- Will tolerate the SLP touching the face
- Will increase sensory awareness and organization
- Will increase midline orientation
- Will increase tone in the buccal and labial musculature
- Will increase upper lip mobility
- Will increase lip rounding
- Will increase jaw strength

- Will increase tongue retraction
- Will improve jaw grading
- Will improve jaw/lip dissociation

1. **Massage:** Start at the temporomandibular joint (TMJ) and provide firm, elongated massage to the corners of Sean's lips, alongside the nostrils into the insertion of the upper lip, and from under the nostrils into the upper lip. Do each set 4-5 times. Vary the sensory input and incorporate into daily living activities.

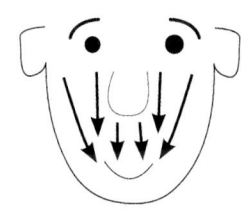

Sensory Suggestions:

- Bare hands – prior to meals, play
- Lotion – after bath
- Wet/dry washcloths – before/after meals, after bath
- Warm/cold washcloths – bath time
- Textured bean bags – play
- Vibration – play

This will increase sensory awareness and organization, encourage midline orientation and facilitate increased cheek, and upper lip mobility.

2. **Tap-n-Tone:** Provide firm, rhythmic tapping from the TMJ to the corners of the lips and on the surface of the lips to the beat of a favorite finger play activity or nursery rhyme.

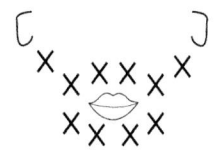

This will provide sensory input and tone to the buccal and labial musculature.

Appendix E: Sample Report

3. **Cheek Resistance with Slide:**

   A. Present the Z-vibe® yellow preefer head in Sean's cheek and stretch out.

   B. Slide the tool to the corner of Sean's lips (like you are taking a lollipop out of his mouth) as you instruct him to kiss.

   C. As the tool comes to midline instruct Sean to do a fish kiss.

   Do each "set" 5 times.

4. **Upper Lip Stretch:** You can do this exercise with a Z-vibe® yellow preefer tip. Start under Sean's top lip and roll from the corner of the lip to midline. Stop. Repeat on the opposite side. Do each "set" 4-5 times.

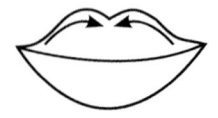

   This will provide sensory input and increased upper lip mobility.

5. **Cheek Toning/Lip Rounding:** Present the rounded end of the Jiggler between his lips. Provide jaw/cheek support as needed to facilitate lip rounding. Model a [w] sound and encourage Sean to imitate. Repeat 10 times or as he will tolerate.

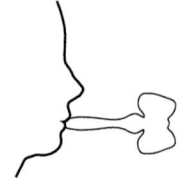

   This will provide sensory input, facilitate increased tone in the cheeks, and encourage lip rounding.

6. **Bilateral Tongue Hugs:** You will need two Z-vibes® small, square, green heads for this exercise. Present the Z-vibes® bilaterally along the lateral borders of the tongue. Stroke firmly to the tongue tip. Repeat 5 times/2 sets.

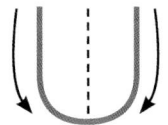

This will increase elongation through the lateral borders of the tongue and facilitate a tongue tip.

7. **Bilateral Chewy Tubes:** (You will need two yellow and two red Chewy Tubes® for this exercise).

   A. Present the yellow Chewy Tubes® bilaterally and perpendicular to the lateral molar ridges at the insertion of the back molars. Instruct Sean to do 10 slow, graded, repetitive bites. You may need to provide a visual model. Provide jaw support as demonstrated.

   B. Repeat with the red tubes.

This will increase jaw strength, jaw symmetry, tongue retraction, and graded movement.

Feeding:

1. **Spoon Feeding:** Use a vibrating spoon for purees. Turn the spoon sideways, contacting the corners of Sean's lips. Tilt the spoon slightly if you observe him biting the spoon.

This will encourage lip closure and tongue retraction.

2. **Fork Feeding:** Use a cocktail-type/narrow fork for this exercise. Cut food into "Cheerio®- sized" pieces and spear on the fork. Present the fork upside down and perpendicular to the lateral molar ridge. Alternate the side you present the fork on.

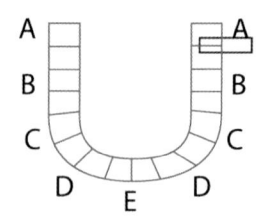

This will increase jaw grading, tongue retraction and a lateral chew.

3. **Chewing Hierarchy:** Follow the directions on the protocol for Chewing Hierarchy level #1 using a stick-shaped bolus. Alternate sides and repeat.

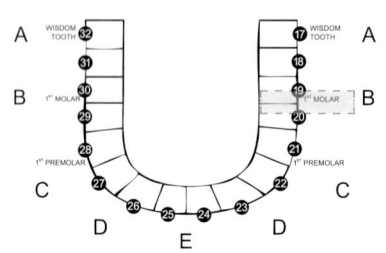

This will encourage a lateral chew, jaw grading and tongue retraction.

4. **Straw Drinking:** Sean should be drinking from TalkTools® straw #1 cut to 1 inch above the animal head /lip block. Over the next several weeks soak the top of the straw in hot water and trim above the animal head/lip block. Eventually there should only be ¼ inch of straw above the animal head/lip block. Encourage him to do single sips.

This will increase lip rounding and tongue retraction.

Re-evaluation: Four months.

LORI L. OVERLAND,
M.S., CCC-SLP, C/NDT

Lori L. Overland

ROBYN MERKEL-WALSH,
M.A., CCC-SLP

Robyn M. Walsh MA CCC-SLP

REFERENCES

American Speech-Language-Hearing Association (ASHA). (2009). *Roles of speech language pathologists in swallowing and feeding disorders* [Technical Report]. Retrieved from www.asha.org/policy.

Apel, K. (1999). Checks and balances: Keeping the science in our profession. *Language, Speech, and Hearing Services in the Schools*, 30, 99-108.

Arvedson, J., & Brodksy, L. (2001). *Pediatric swallowing and feeding: Assessment and management* (2nd ed.). Albany, NY: Singular.

Bahr, D. (2001). *Oral motor assessment and treatment: Ages and stages.* Boston, MA: Allyn & Bacon.

Bahr, D. (2010). *Nobody ever told me (or my mother) that! Everything from bottles and breathing to healthy speech development.* Arlington, TX: Sensory World.

Bahr, D., & Rosenfeld-Johnson, S. (2010). Treatment of children with speech oral placement disorders (OPDs): A paradigm emerges. *Communication Disorders Quarterly,* 31, 131-138.

Balzola F, et al. (2006). Beneficial behavioral effects of IBD therapy and gluten/casein-free diet in an Italian cohort of patients with autistic enterocolitis followed over one year. *Gastroenterology*, 130(4), S1364 A-21.

Balzola, F., Barbon, V., Repici, A., & Rizzetto, M. (2005). Panenteric IBD-like disease in a patient with regressive autism shown for the first time by the wireless capsule enteroscopy: Another piece in the jigsaw of this gut-brain syndrome? *American Journal of Gastroenterology*, 979-981.

Bartlett, D., & Werner, J. (2006). Enteral feeding tubes and gastric decompression tubes. Retrieved from http://www.radiographicceu.com/article24.html.

Boshart, C. (1999). *Oral-facial illustrations and reference guide.* Montgomery, TX: Speech Dynamics, Inc. Available from http://www.speechdynamics.com/oral-facial-illustrations-and-reference-guide?page=shop.product_details&flypage=flypage.tpl&product_id=5&category_id=3.

Boshart, C. (2001). *Progressive oral sensory-motor therapy: Paradigm and procedures.* Temecula, CA.

Boyle, C., Decoufle, P., & Yeargin-Allsopp, M. (1994). *Prevalence and health impact of developmental disabilities in US children. Pediatrics*, 93, 399-403.

Clark, H., & Osrty, D. (2005). *Contributions to speech motor control. American Speech and Hearing Association.* San Diego, CA.

Cole, S., & Lanham, J. (2011). Failure to thrive: An update. Retrieved June 30, 2012 from http://www.aafp.org/afp/2011/0401/p829.html.

Dorfman, K. (n.d.). How nutrition impacts muscle tone. Retrieved July 11 from www.kellydorfman.com

Eig, J. (2002). The popular spill-free vessel suddenly comes under fire for speech slurs, cavities. *Arizona Daily Star*. Retrieved from http://azstarnet.com/.

Fasano, A. (2011). Interview with Dr. Alession Fasano, Part 1: should anyone eat gluten? Retrieved on 7/12/12 from www.tenderfoodie.com/blog/211/12/19.

Fedorak, R., & Madsen, K. (2004). Probiotics and the management of inflammatory bowel disease. *Inflammatory Bowel Disease,* 10(3), 286.

Fisher, A., Murray, E., & Bundy, A. (Eds.). (1991). *Sensory integration: Theory and practice.* Philadelphia, PA: F.A. Davis.

Food Allergy and Anaphylaxis Network (FAAN). (2012). Food allergy facts and statistics for the US. Retrieved June 1, 2012 from http://www.foodallergy.org/files/FoodAllergyFactsandStatistics.pdf.

Food and Drug Administration (FDA). (n.d.) Avoiding drug interaction. Retrieved November 8, 2011 from http://www.fda.gov/forconsumers/consumerupdates/ucm096386.htm.

Fucile, S., Gisel, E., & Lau, C. (2002). Oral stimulation accelerates the transition from tube to oral feeding in preterm infants. *Journal of Pediatrics*, 141, 230-236.

Genna, C.W. (2012). *Supporting sucking in breast feeding infants,* (2nd ed.). Burlington, MA: Jones and Bartlett Learning.

Gonzalez, L., Lopez, K., Navarro, D., Negron, L., Flores, L., Rodriguez, R., Martinez, M., & Sabra, A. (n.d.). Endoscopic and histological characteristics of the digestive mucosa in autistic children with gastrointestinal symptoms. *Arch Venez Pueric Pediatr.*, 69(1), 19-25.

Gottschall, E. (1994). *Breaking the Vicious Cycle* (Revised edition). The Kirkton Press.

Green, J., Moore, C., Ruark, J., Rodda, P., Morvee, W., & VanWitzenburg, M. (1997). Development of chewing in children from 12 to 48 months: Longitudinal study of EMG patterns. *Journal of Neurophysiology,* 77, 2704-2716.

Hanson, M., Mason, R. (2003). *Oral facial mycology: international perspectives.* Springfield, IL: Charles C. Thomas Publishing Inc.

Hassall, E. (2005). Decisions in diagnosing and managing chronic gastroesophageal reflux disease in children. *Journal of Pediatrics,* 146(3), 3-12.

Higgenbotham. (2010). Effectiveness and safety of PPIs in infantile GERD. *Annals of Pharmacotherapy*, 44(3).

Homan, M., Baldassano, R., & Mamula, P. (2005). Managing complicated Crohn's disease in children and adolescents. *Nature Clinical Practice Gastroenterology & Hepatology*, 2(12), 572-9.

Horvath, K., et al. (1999). Gastrointestinal abnormalities in children with autistic disorder. *Journal of Pediatrics*, 135(5), 559-63.

Horvath, K., & Perman, J. (2002). Autism and gastrointestinal symptoms. *Current Gastroenterology Reports*, 4(3), 251-8.

Huang, R., Forbes, D., et al. (2002). Feed thickener for newborn infants with gastro-oesophageal reflux. *Cochrane Database of Systematic Reviews*, 3.

Knox, J. (2008). The use of rice cereal as an alternative thickener in commonly used pediatric fluids: a feasibility study: A summary of findings. Retrieved July 10 from http://nutrition.otago.ac.nz/__data/assets/file/0003/4755/DTP_JKnox_SoF.pdf.

Kuddo, T., & Nelson, K. (2003). How common are gastrointestinal disorders in children with autism? *Current Opinions in Pediatrics*, 15(3), 339-343.

McEachin, J., Smith, T., & Lovaas, O. (1993). Long-term outcome for children with autism who received early intensive behavioral treatment. *American Journal on Mental Retardation*, 97(4), 359-372.

March of Dimes. (2012). *Prematurity campaign*. Retrieved From http://www.marchofdimes.com/mission/prematurity_indepth.html.

Marshalla, Pam (2007). Oral motor techniques are not new. *Oral Motor Institute*, 1 (1). Availabale from www.oralmotorinstitute.org.

Marshalla, P. (2012). Horns, whistles, bite blocks, and straws: A review of tools/objects used in articulation therapy by Van Riper and other traditional therapists. *Oral Motor Institute*, 4(2). Available from www.oralmotorinstitute.org.

Merkel-Walsh, R., & Rosenfeld-Johnson, S. (2003). Connections between tongue placement and dental alignment. *ADVANCE for Speech-Language Pathologists & Audiologists*, 13(36), 9.

Merkel-Walsh, R. (2001). *Tongue thrust therapy: An oral motor approach to diagnosis and treatment* [DVD]. Talk Tools Innovative Therapists International.

Merkel-Walsh, R. (2012). *Solving the puzzle of autism: using tactile therapy techniques* [Live Seminar]. Talk Tools Innovative Therapists International.

Merkel-Walsh , R. (2012). *Assessment of oral placement disorders: Structure, tone and function* [Webinar]. Available from www.AAPPSPA.org.

Merkel, R. (2002). *Systematic intervention for lingual elevation*. Tucson, AZ: Talk Tools Innovative Therapists International.

Moore, C., & Ruark, J. (1996). Does speech emerge from earlier appearing oral motor behaviors? *Journal of Speech and Hearing Research*, 39, 1034-1047.

Moore, C., Smith, A., & Ringel, R. (1988). Task-specific organization of activity in human jaw muscles. *Journal of Speech and Hearing Research*, 31, 670-680.

Morris, S., & Klein, M. (1987). *Pre-feeding skills: A comprehensive resource for feeding development* (2nd ed.). San Antonio, TX: Therapy Skill Builders.

Morris, S., & Klein, M. (2000). *Pre-feeding skills* (2nd ed). San Antonio, TX: Therapy Skill Builders.

National Institution of Neurological Diseases and Stroke (NINDS). (2008). *Post Stroke Rehabilitation Brochure* [PDF document]. Retrieved from http://www.ninds.nih.gov/disorders/stroke/poststrokerehab.htm.

Orenstein, S., Izadnia, F., & Kahn, S. (1999). Gastrointestinal reflux disease in children. *Gastroenterol Clinical North America*, 28, 947-969.

Osterweil, Neil. (2012). Foods that may worsen pollen allergies. Retrieved on May 5, 2012 from http://www.webmd.com/allergies/features/oral-allergy-syndrome-foods.

O'Sullivan, S. (2007). Examination of motor function: Motor control and motor learning. In S.B. O'Sullivan, & T. J. Schmitz (Eds). Physical rehabilitation (5th ed.). Philadelphia, PA: F. A. Davis Company.

Overland, L. (2001). Food for thought. *ADVANCE for Speech-Language Pathologists & Audiologists*.

Overland, L. (2011). *A sensory-motor approach to feeding. Perspectives on Swallowing and Swallowing Disorders* (Dysphagia), 20, 60-64.

Palmer, B. (2001). Frenums, tongue-tie, ankyloglossia. Retrieved July 10 from www.brianpalmerdds.com.

Pierce, R. (1980). The role of oral motor therapy in speech pathology. *International Journal of Orofacial Myology*, 6.

Reilly, S., Douglas, J., & Oates, J. (Eds.) (2004). *Evidence-Based Practice in Speech Pathology*. London: Whurr Publishers.

Rocha, A., Moreira, M., Pimenta, H., Ramos, J., & Lucena, S. (2007). A Randomized study of the efficacy of sensory-motor-oral stimulation and non-nutritive sucking in very low birth weight infant. *Early Human Development*, 83(6), 385-388.

Roche, W., Eicher, P., Martorana, P., Berkowitz, M., Petronchak, J., Dzioba, J., & Vitello, L. (2011). An oral, motor, medical, and behavioral approach to pediatric feeding and swallowing disorders: An interdisciplinary model. *Perspectives on Swallowing and Swallowing Disorders* (Dysphagia), 20, 65-74.

Rosenfeld-Johnson, S. (1997). The Oral-Motor Myths of Down Syndrome. *ADVANCE for Speech-Language Pathologists & Audiologists*.

Rosenfeld-Johnson, S. (2004) Proceedings from 26th World Congress of the International Association of
Logopedics and Phoniatrics: *Oral-Motor Exercises for Speech Clarity*. Brisbane: Australia.

Rosenfeld-Johnson, S. (2006) Proceedings from International Down Syndrome Conference: *Safe Feeding and Prevention of Ear Infections in Down Syndrome*. Vancouver, BC: Canada.

Sjögreen, L., Tulinius, M., Kiliaridis, S., & Lohmander, A. (2010). The effect of lip strengthening exercises in children and adolescents with myotonic dystrophy type 1. *International Journal of Pediatric Otorhinolaryngology*, 74(10), 1126-1134.

Sackett, D. Rosenberg, W., Gray, J., Haynes, R., & Richardson, W. (1996). Evidence-based medicine: What it is and what it isn't. *British Medical Journal*, 312, 71-72.

Sackett, D., Straus, S., Richardson, W., Rosenberg, W., & Haynes, R. (2000). *Evidence-Based Medicine: How to Practice and Teach EBM*. Edinburgh: Churchill Livingstone.

Shumway-Cook, A., & Woollacott, M.H. (2001). *Motor control: Theory and Practical Applications* (2nd ed.). Philadelphia: Lippincott Williams & Wilkins.

Shrader and Associates. (2011). Simply thick recall & necrotizing enterocolitis (NEC) connection. Retrieved from http://www.shraderlaw.com/blog/2011/06/24/simply-thick-necrotizing-enterocolitis-nec/.

Strand, E., & Sullivan, M. (2001). Evidence-based practice guidelines for dysarthria: Management for velopharyngeal function. *Journal of Medical Speech-Language Pathology*, 9, 257-274.

Trelka, J., & Hooker, B. (2004). Specific Carbohydrate Dietary Trial: Understanding the Effectiveness of a Specific Carbohydrate. Dietary Intervention In Autistic Children. *uclbs news*.

Valicenti-McDermott, M., McVicar, K., Rapin, I., Wershil, BK., Cohen, H., & Shinnar, S. (2006). Frequency of gastrointestinal symptoms in children with autistic spectrum disorders and association with family history of autoimmune disease. *Journal of Developmental & Behavioral Pediatrics*, 27(2), S128-36.

Valicenti-McDermott, M., McVicar, K., Cohen, H., Wershil, B., & Shinnar, S. (2008). Gastrointestinal symptoms in children with an autism spectrum disorder and language regression. *Pediatric Neurology*, 39(6),392-8.

Toomey, K., & Sundseth Ross, E. (2011). *SOS approach to feeding*. Perspectives on Swallowing and Swallowing Disorders (Dysphagia), 20, 82-87.